MW00761173

COSMICALLY CHIC

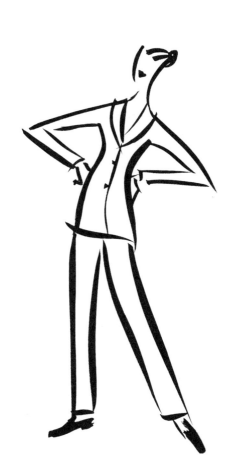

COSMICALLY CHIC

DISCOVERING YOUR FASHION STYLE

THROUGH ASTROLOGY

GREG POLKOSNIK

Andrews McMeel
Publishing

Kansas City

*Cosmically Chic: Discovering Your Fashion Style
through Astrology* copyright © 2000 by Greg Polkosnik.
All rights reserved. Printed in the United States of America.
No part of this book may be used or reproduced in any
manner whatsoever without written permission except
in the case of reprints in the context of reviews.
For information, write Andrews McMeel Publishing,
an Andrews McMeel Universal company,
4520 Main Street, Kansas City, Missouri 64111.

00 01 02 03 04 RDC 10 9 8 7 6 5 4 3 2 1

Library of Congress Cataloging-in-Publication Data

Polkosnik, Greg.
 Cosmically chic : discovering your fashion style through
 astrology / Greg Polkosnik.
     p. cm.
 ISBN 0-7407-1017-6 (pbk.)
     1. Astrology. 2. Clothing and dress—Miscellanea. I. Title.
BF1729.W64 P65 2000
646'.34—dc21   00-033152

Book design by Holly Camerlinck
Illustrations by Sharon Watts

——————— **Attention: Schools and Businesses** ———————

Andrews McMeel books are available at quantity discounts with
bulk purchase for educational, business, or sales promotional use.
For information, please write to: Special Sales Department,
Andrews McMeel Publishing, 4520 Main Street,
Kansas City, Missouri 64111.

This book is dedicated to my friend Marjie.
Now she has no excuse not to dress better.

COSMICALLY CHIC

CONTENTS

WHAT IS COSMIC CHIC?

In astrology the sun represents the essence of your spirit. Whether you are an Aries, a Pisces, or any other zodiac sign, your sun sign is the material that makes you who you are. It is the fabric of your being. You cannot change the material you are made from, and you cannot change your sun sign. The sun endows you with your sense of self-expression. While you may be able to change the manner in which you create your image, your sense of self-expression is already fabricated. For this reason you must learn to express an image that is harmonious with the fabric you are made from—a cosmically chic image, to be precise.

Many astrologers believe the rising sign has the greatest impact on the creation of an individual's self-image. However, the rising sign does not govern one's sense of self-expression. Instead, it determines the manner of expression, and it alters the way you behave. Your rising sign also affects the way you wear your clothes. It has more to do with your physical demeanor and your poise than with your sense of self. Your rising sign can be compared to a mask that you wear in order to comfortably express yourself to others. But it can hinder your sense of self-expression by concealing who you really are.

There are other factors that can affect the way you express yourself. The placement of the sun in your chart can affect whether you feel the influence of your sun sign more than your rising sign, or vice versa. A particularly weak sun can cause you to disregard the influence of the sun entirely in favor of your rising sign. If you have a weak sun placement, perhaps you feel more comfortable dressing in the style of your rising sign (any good astrologer can tell you where the sun is placed in your chart). The placement of Venus in your chart also can affect the way you dress. Venus rules your aesthetic sense. A poorly placed Venus can mean that you have been endowed with bad taste. A well-placed Venus is often evident in the charts of people who adore fashion. Nevertheless, your sun sign is intrinsically concerned with self-expression, and you should not overlook its influence upon the way you dress.

You should never overlook the importance of fashion, either. If you dress in a cosmically chic style that expresses the essence of your being, you will feel better about yourself. Fashion is often rejected by its harshest critics as a superficial pursuit that exploits the anxieties of insecure individuals. Nothing could be further from the truth. Fashion affords all of us the chance to be more confident about the way we look. The self-confidence that you derive from being pleased with your appearance cannot be dismissed as superficial. The feeling that you get from looking good is good for your spirit. If astrology plays a role in your spiritual beliefs, then fashion astrology can be good for your spirit, too.

HOW TO USE THIS BOOK

The problem with sun sign astrology is that it characterizes entire groups of people with broad generalizations. Sun sign astrology may tell you that Virgos find Capricorns sexually attractive. However, the success of a relationship is determined more accurately by assessing the placement of Venus and Mars in a chart comparison. Sun sign astrology also may tell you that Geminis make great writers. But the position of Mercury in a chart offers more insight into how effectively an individual communicates. Sun sign astrology gives astrology a bad name because it deals in clichés.

Nevertheless, certain clichés exist about each sign for a reason. If there never was a bullheaded Taurus or a crabby Cancer, these clichés wouldn't endure. People often express themselves in a negative manner, and negative behavior can be much more memorable than positive conduct. For this reason, each chapter of *Cosmically Chic* begins with a brief discussion of the characteristics that define a particular sign—including all the clichés.

The fashion advice that follows is meant to be adapted to the type of woman you are. Each section should have some relevance in the context of your own life. The suggestions are general enough to allow you to adapt them to your own age, race, or body type. The advice is also rather "trend neutral," so you can refer back to it time and time again. Designer labels are recommended for each sign, but only to provide you with an idea of your sign's signature style. Unfortunately, many great fashion designers are not mentioned in the text simply because they have capricious natures themselves and don't fit comfortably under a certain sign. The celebrity profiles are meant to serve as illustrations only, and they are not intended to insult anyone. In fact, there are far more examples of well-dressed women in this book than examples of poorly dressed women.

When you have read your own chapter, I encourage you to read the rest of the book. There is much more to *Cosmically Chic* than fashion advice. Each chapter provides insights into the way the sun manifests its power in a zodiac sign. But aside from providing you with information about the signs themselves, this book can be a lot of fun. After reading each chapter you may find yourself looking at people in a different way, trying to guess their astrological signs on the basis of their appearance. Don't be afraid to ask someone "What's your sign?" in order to prove or disprove your assertions. You shouldn't be ashamed to believe in astrology. If you learn to use astrology in the manner in which it was intended, it can open up a world of possibilities for you. Astrology's most vocal detractors dismiss the study because of the inaccuracy of daily horoscopes. But horoscopes are often written for entertainment value alone. I do hope you find this book entertaining, but I also hope that when you put it down you have learned something about astrology. I hope you come to understand exactly how the sun makes you who you are.

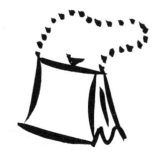

ARIES
THE RAM

March 21-April 20

WHAT MAKES YOU
AN ARIES

Picture the zodiac as a circle with no beginning and no end, no first place and no last place. In this cosmic cycle each sign gradually blends into the next just as naturally as the seasons flow into one another. Now imagine how disappointing this image is to the Aries woman. As an Aries you know that you don't like to be anything but first. Even when "first place" is merely a starting point, rather than a reflection of some first-rate performance, being first makes you feel like you're special. But this preoccupation with being first can be a sort of double-edged sword. On the positive side, you can be both an initiator and an innovator, forging ahead into uncharted territory and discovering things that the rest of us never would have found. However, your attention span can be remarkably short. You may be a great starter, Aries, but you are also a terrible finisher. Many of you abandon what you've started simply because you've lost interest in it.

The driving force behind your desire to be in first place is your ruling planet, Mars. In Roman mythology Mars was the god of war. Mars always jumped headfirst into everything he did, letting his testosterone-driven impulses supersede his rational thought processes. Like the mythological character it is named after, the planet Mars symbolizes energy and aggression. Consequently, Mars endows all Aries individuals with these qualities. This probably is not what every Aries woman wants to hear, but does it come as much of a surprise to you? You know it is this combative energy that pushes you forward and makes you feel the need to dominate those around you. Mars can give you the swaggering bravado and cocksure attitude of a teenager, but it also can give you an aggressive nature and a reckless disregard for others. Unfocused Martian energy can be a terribly destructive force, both selfish and cruel. Fortunately, reckless Mars is just a single aspect of what makes you an Aries.

Like Leo and Sagittarius, Aries is a fire sign. It is also a cardinal sign. The element of fire is what gives you your confidence. Likewise, the cardinal quality gives you a directness in thought and speech, as well as the focus that helps you rein in the worst of what Martian energy has to offer. When the influence of Mars is combined with the fire element and the cardinal quality, typical Aries characteristics become evident. If you express these characteristics in a positive manner, you can be honest, single-minded, energetic, bold, and passionate. If you express these characteristics negatively, you can be brusque, conceited, frantic, reckless, and impulsive. Since you are often more concerned with your own opinion of yourself than with what others think of you, you must try to cultivate those positive characteristics. By doing so you can develop a less self-centered persona to present to the world. Once you accomplish this, Aries, you will find that others can be just as interested in you as you are in yourself. This is important to you because you really don't like to be left alone. Therefore, in order to attract the kinds of relationships you desire, you should possess a personal style that others find irresistible. You need to draw people into your world with an alluring personal style, rather than scare them off with a reckless appearance and an aggressive demeanor.

YOUR KEYWORD

The keyword every Aries woman should keep in mind when creating her personal style is *impact*. Your Aries fire is like a flame on the fuse of a stick of dynamite. As the flame dances along the fuse, it crackles and pops, creating a commotion in the moment itself. Yet there is only one direction the flame may move: forward. Behind the flame there is no fuel left to sustain it, and therefore nothing of value. Like that flame, fiery Aries women thrive in the here and now. You are at your most powerful when you recognize that it is in your nature to focus on the immediate. The best-dressed Aries women appear stylish because they are forward-looking: They keep up-to-date, and they never look to the past for inspiration. Consequently, you ought to possess a personal style that is contemporary. You must let everyone know exactly what is fashionable from the moment you walk into a room. Keep your mind on the future, Aries, and you'll be amazed at the impact you have upon others.

YOUR THREE RULES TO DRESS BY

1: Simplify

Aries is a very uncomplicated sign. As such, you will always be at your best by following this advice: Be yourself. Keep your wardrobe simple, and keep your closet stocked with the few basic items you believe genuinely reflect what you're about. Avoid complicated garments and meticulous detailing. Well-constructed clothing in solid colors and simple geometric prints will hold your interest much longer than anything fussy or ornate. Good tailoring is also extremely important to Aries women. Since your clothes are just an externalization of the way you're feeling on the inside, you'll want them to fit perfectly to avoid misrepresenting yourself to others. If you don't think your wardrobe is shouting "This is me!" to everyone around you, then you need to get back to basics. So clean out your closet, slim down your wardrobe, and simplify, simplify, simplify.

2: Modernize

You, Aries, are infamous for living in the moment. Unfortunately, much of what the fashion world has to offer you is based on a romantic idealization of the past, and you don't do retro well. You should thank your lucky stars that there are a few designers who embrace the future and provide the innovative, contemporary clothing you were born to wear. However, you do need a few words of caution regarding your fashion-forward orientation. First, you should try to avoid terribly trendy styles, because you may lose interest in being a fashion pioneer even before the trend has passed. Your lack of staying power can be your biggest weakness. Also, don't shun the classics because they bore you, but embrace them because of what made them classic: timeless simplicity. Sleek, modern interpretations of the classics are what you'll always carry off best.

3: Androgynize

As mentioned before, Aries is ruled by Mars, the most masculine planet. This can give Aries women a sort of manly cast, which they may or may not feel comfortable with. On the one hand, you could feel a natural inclination to wear rather masculine styles. On the other hand, you might overcompensate with ruffles and flowers, or with lace and pastels, just to disguise the fact that your hormones seem to be a little out of balance. However, if you are living—or dressing—in either of these scenarios, you are making a big mistake. Aries women need to dress as if they are straddling the center of the gender spectrum. Not too boyish, not too girlish. Not too rugged, not too cutesy. You must learn to strike a balance between the masculine and feminine elements in your closet. A little androgyny may not only make you feel more comfortable in your clothing but also make you feel more comfortable in your own skin.

SPECIFICS: WHAT TO WEAR

✧ To get the impact you desire out of your clothes, wear red. Red is Mars's color. It is vibrant, aggressive, and attention-getting. Except for funerals, you can wear red absolutely anywhere. It's almost impossible to go wrong with your signature color, Aries. Winter, spring, summer, or fall, red is one of the few colors that works great year-round.

✧ Woven fabrics suit you better than knits. Except for the shaggiest tweeds, men's suiting fabrics will appeal to you, too. Avoid cute fabrics like gingham, seersucker, or eyelet. You're no farmer's daughter, so don't try to dress like one.

✧ Red is one of the only bright colors that can be worn as a neutral, matching almost any color it is paired with. But there are many other neutral colors that suit you well. Black, gray, navy, and beige all are good choices for you.

✧ A little red dress can be your little black dress.

✧ Monochromatic color schemes appeal to your love of simplicity. Also, single-color garments are especially attractive to your minimalistic sense of style. The fewer colors you wear, the better you look.

✧ Minimalism itself comes and goes like any fashion trend, but simplicity is always in fashion for you. Don't complicate your life by jumping on the trend bandwagon.

✧ As the modernist of the zodiac, you often feel left out of the retro trends. However, 1940s femme fatale is a classic Aries look.

✧ Avoid black leather, unless you're looking for work as a dominatrix.

✧ Go shopping with your friends. Your brutal honesty can save them from making terrible mistakes.

✧ Aries women excel at separates dressing. Fashion magazines frequently demonstrate how a few basic separates can carry you through a season or two when mixed and matched appropriately. It is the simple nature of the coordinates selected for these layouts that allows for the creation of the final product: a wardrobe. The clothes that work best in this context never seem too formal, nor do they appear too casual. Within the middle ground of these styles is your own look: a simple, straightforward chic.

✦ You probably don't spend a lot of money on clothes. Most Aries women like to spread their money around, and they usually don't focus their spending on a particular area, such as their wardrobes. But when you do spend a lot of money, it is likely that you spend it on something foolish, since impulse control can be difficult for someone who truly lives in the moment. Control yourself, Aries. Always think twice before you open your wallet.

✦ Chances are you have a penchant for pants. While it is possible that you wear skirts just as often as anyone else, Aries definitely is the sign that "wears the pants" in the zodiac. Use this fact to your advantage. Pantsuits are an ideal Aries outfit.

✦ Remember that you do have a tendency to wear clothes a little on the masculine side, so choose pieces wisely. Avoid jackets with shoulder pads when you think you can do without them. The actress Joan Crawford was an Aries, and people remember her infamous shoulder pads to this day.

✦ Because of its association with warlike Mars, Aries rules over the military. Designers often add military elements to their collections, and you can use these elements to your advantage. However, be careful not to go over the top: Don't dress like you're ready for combat.

✦ A pair of sleek military-style boots, or a tailored red coat with a touch of military hardware can go a long way for you. In fact, if you can only buy one piece to improve your wardrobe for any season, a great red coat is a terrific choice.

✦ You may find safari-inspired clothing appealing. As well, nautical looks inspired by the Navy and Marine Corps are a sure bet for you. Just remember that striking a balance between masculine and feminine influences is your biggest fashion challenge, and militaristic styles can be a bit risky.

✦ When choosing what to wear you must also consider your attitude. As mentioned before, nothing pleases you more than knowing that you are the master of whatever you do. But many Aries women adopt a queen-of-the-hill attitude without putting in the effort it takes to sit on that throne. No one likes a windbag, especially when that windbag is all hot air. If you are going to boast that you are dressed better than everyone else, then you ought to dress better than everyone else. Arrogance is even more loathsome when you don't live up to the high standards you expect of others. Aries women thrive on the adulation of the crowd, so you need to be especially careful that you don't drive everyone away with an overcritical attitude. If you're not careful, you could wake up one day to find yourself alone and miserable—not to mention badly dressed.

WHO TO WEAR

The best minimalist designers have earned that title by presenting collections always in tune with your simple Aries style. The current king of minimalism is Calvin Klein. From his clothes on the runway to his spare print and television ads, and even the designs of his signature fragrance bottles, Calvin Klein has presented a clear, consistent vision of what he believes style is. Uncomplicated and never fussy, his modern designs are a perfect match for your straightforward style. Fortunately, his clothes are available in a few lines, one of which likely falls into your price range. Among the Calvin Klein signature label, CK2, Calvin Klein Jeans, and the countless knockoff versions of his clothes, there are a myriad of choices.

Another line that appeals to your fashion sensibilities is Donna Karan's DKNY. Donna Karan, like Calvin Klein, is a modernist, but her clothes often have a more opulent or sophisticated look. The DKNY label, however, is more youthful and much sportier than her signature collection. This streetwise line should suit you well. Michael Kors also designs a signature label that is simple, sexy, and beautiful, but you might want to avoid the slightly more showy clothing he designs for the French label Celine. There is an understated elegance to the collections of Karan, Kors, and Klein. In fact, many of the New York designers' collections seem to be geared toward a rather understated consumer. Most successful American designers focus on sportswear, and they usually let the European designers worry about showing off. For this reason, North American Aries women should have little difficulty in finding labels that complement their uncomplicated style. For instance, many designers' secondary collections work beautifully for you. This is because most secondary collections consist of simplified, less expensive versions of the signature garments. You'll also find that plenty top-of-the-line department store labels suit you well. Just remember, it is inevitable for you to grow tired of your clothes, regardless of who designed them. You crave change, so you need to buy outfits that won't drain your checking account, since you know they will be replaced sooner rather than later.

WHAT TO AVOID

When an Aries woman is badly dressed, it is usually because she cannot accept the truth of her androgynous nature. Her attempts to make herself more feminine are disastrous. Ruffles, bows, fringe, lace, ribbons, sequins, appliqués, and so on can be bad news for you. Don't complicate your wardrobe with excessive detail. Avoid designers who make "pretty" clothes, because they can make you look as if you're wearing Christmas wrap. You like to command attention, but not the kind of attention that type of clothing will attract. A Valentino dress, for instance, can be a work of art, but it likely would make you feel like a festive holiday centerpiece or a parade float. Sexy, attention-getting clothes, like the kind Todd Oldham used to design for

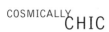

his signature label, are also a bad bet for you. The same can be said about the marvelously girlish clothes of Betsey Johnson and the styles of many other "cheesecake" designers.

You could go, however, in the opposite direction and dress like a sloppy teenage boy. Tracksuits, baseball caps, sports logo gear, and other boyish looks surely will get you noticed, but mostly by those who are laughing behind your back. It is essential for you to realize that the Aries tendency to live in the moment should never manifest itself as a careless, tactless, or juvenile attitude. Being appropriately dressed for whatever the occasion demands will get you a lot further than breaking rules the rest of us have to live—and dress—by.

HAIR AND MAKEUP

Each sign rules a specific area of the body. Aries holds rulership over the top of the head, the face, and especially the eyes. This is important for you to recognize because it is likely that your eyes are uncommonly expressive. You probably don't hold back a great deal emotionally, but chances are you couldn't: People know what you're feeling when they look into your eyes. The film legend Bette Davis was an Aries, and someone wrote a song about her eyes. So make the most of what you've got, and learn to use eye makeup to your advantage. Buy some fashion magazines and note the trends. Update your colors and application techniques frequently. Don't be afraid of a little drama either—just go ahead and have some fun. And, by all means, allow yourself to look like a girl. Makeup is the key you need to escape from the masculine influence of Mars. Although simplicity works best for you in most cases, your eyes are like a canvas on which you can express your creativity. For the rest of your face *clean, easy,* and *uncomplicated* are three words to keep in mind when buying and applying cosmetics. As well, remember to downplay the makeup on your cheeks and lips so that they don't draw attention away from those stunning Aries eyes.

As far as your hair is concerned, try to wear an uncomplicated style that is easy to maintain. Fussing and primping in front of the mirror are things a restless Aries woman rarely finds pleasure in. You have a short attention span and a lot of better things to do. So take this advice: Shell out whatever it costs for a great hairstylist. Find someone who can give you a good low-maintenance cut that is easy to keep up-to-date. You ought to have a contemporary hairstyle, but be careful of trendy looks and boyish cuts. A simple hair clip or barrette will work much better for you than a lot of hardware. Also, be wary of long hair: It can be way too much work for you. Color changes may help you to stay on fashion's cutting edge, but be careful because many of you hair-obsessed Aries women also like to perm your hair. Keep in mind that too many chemical processes occurring simultaneously can be disastrous for hair. Avoid problems by choosing either the new color or the perm. You don't have to rush into everything at once, Aries. Learn to appreciate the fact that you can change your mind—and your hair—the next time.

ACCESSORIES

Wear little or no jewelry. Keep it simple. Your look is modern and simple, but often you desire an edginess from fashion that you can quickly grow out of. Spending your hard-earned money on wardrobe pieces that don't get worn is foolish, and you know it's foolish because you've done it. However, there is a solution to this problem that will kill two birds with one stone, satisfying both your need to seek out new fashion trends and your subsequent abandonment of things you've grown weary of. Aries women should collect a wardrobe of inexpensive, fashionable sunglasses. Once again, Aries rules the eyes. By accessorizing the eyes and making sunglasses your jewelry, you can enjoy some of the excitement you desire from fashion without having to waste a ton of your money. Even if you wear prescription glasses, try to use those frames to your advantage. Spend your money on the one object people always notice when they look your way, and if possible don't limit yourself to a single pair.

You need to be especially careful to wear the right shoes. A medium- to high-heeled shoe not only will help you soften your look but may also help you stand up straight. This can give you a little more stature, and it may make your commanding presence that much more compelling. And even though many Aries women despise panty hose, always be sure you are wearing the appropriate hosiery.

Another accessory that is an Aries essential is a good modern purse. Despite the fact that men occasionally carry hand-bags, the purse is still viewed as an effeminate accessory, so carrying a purse can help you to make your look more feminine. You should consider carrying a red purse, too. Louis Vuitton's "Epi" leather line is gorgeous in red. Paloma Picasso's bold signature bags also suit your Aries style. The simplicity of a classic Coach bag may appeal to you also. One good purse that will last you a few seasons is a purchase that you need to make, especially if you are carrying around a dime-store monstrosity or some smelly old gym bag. You were born to carry a fabulous red purse, Aries. It's in the stars. And try on some hats. You'll get a kick out of seeing how they look on you.

SOME ADDITIONAL TIPS TO HELP YOU CREATE YOUR OWN COSMIC STYLE

✦ Paint your nails red and keep them fairly short.

✦ Wear feminine, floral scents when you want to feel more attractive.

✦ Remember that "Casual Friday" does not mean "Sweat Suit Friday."

✦ Don't underestimate the importance of chic, modern undergarments. There are times when a sports bra just won't do.

✦ Wear sleek white satin if you're getting married. Carry a simple bouquet of red roses.

- ✦ Just grin and bear it when you are forced to wear a hideous bridesmaid dress. Take it in stride, Aries.
- ✦ When you are stressed out, a good facial will do wonders for you.
- ✦ Simple, elegant red satin pajamas will go far in your boudoir.
- ✦ If you're feeling adventurous, change your eye color with some colored contact lenses.
- ✦ A sporty, one-piece swimsuit is the style for you.

A FEW WOMEN WHO— FOR BETTER OR WORSE— EXEMPLIFY TRUE ARIES STYLE

Rosie O'Donnell: March 21

Even with a stable of makeup artists, hairstylists, and a personal dresser, the television star Rosie O'Donnell occasionally shows up to host her show dressed in baggy athletic gear. There is a word fashion experts use to describe workout wear worn by people who aren't working out. That word is *ugh*.

Joan Crawford: March 23

The screen legend Joan Crawford was a fiery, radiant beauty in 1932's *Grand Hotel*. Next to Greta Garbo's chiffon-draped, prima-donna character, she appeared refreshingly less feminine and infinitely more sexy. But in 1945's *Mildred Pierce* she was completely upstaged by her manly shoulder pads and stiff hair. Draw your own conclusions.

Diana Ross: March 26

Although the spotlight doesn't shine so brightly anymore on the supreme Miss Ross, she still knows how to make heads turn her way, just like an Aries woman should. Catch her at her stylish best in the audience of the big designers' shows, wearing chic, modern clothes and sunglasses, of course.

Camille Paglia: April 2

There probably is not another woman in the world who is a more typical Aries than the author Camille Paglia. She's brash, energetic, and completely aware that she is not the most delicate creature in the zodiac. She always looks smart in her stylish, well-tailored suits.

Bette Davis: April 5

When she won the Oscar for her title role in *Jezebel* (1938), Bette Davis was an Aries actress portraying a character who acted like an Aries. Shocking society's finest in true Aries fashion, Jezebel attended a ball wearing an entirely inappropriate red dress. Just like Bette Davis, Jezebel knew how to look to make herself the center of attention.

CHAPTER TWO

TAURUS
THE BULL

April 21-May 21

WHAT MAKES YOU A TAURUS

Taurus, you have an image problem. Everyone thinks you're stubborn. But that's not completely true. You might be a little bull-headed sometimes, especially when someone wants you to give up something you truly value. However, that's not really being stubborn. You're always ready to accept others whose viewpoints might be different from your own. You probably reach compromises quite easily, too. In fact, you will normally go out of your way to avoid confrontations, to keep everything harmonious in your little world. Nevertheless, when you fight, you're a force to be reckoned with. This is the Taurus that people remember, and this is why you have an image problem.

You know you're not all that bad, so there has to be a reason why people believe you are. Maybe it's because you're so terribly possessive. You're also defensive, and even a little too lazy. But none of this is your fault, Taurus. You really should blame your ruling planet, Venus. Venus is the mythological goddess of love, beauty, and harmony. She has generously bestowed on you an appreciation for the finer things in life, and a love of pleasure that no other sign can match. As well, she has sharpened your emotional connections with others, helping you to become quite sensitive. She has endowed you with compassion, and she has made you deeply interested in the well-being of everyone around you. However, her influence is not exactly maternal, like the influence of the moon. Instead, it is like that of an affectionate, doting aunt. She is nice, polite, and pretty, and she just wants everyone to get along. It doesn't matter if you don't want to share your toys, or if you go outside to play without cleaning your room first. Everything is okay with her, just as long as you're happy. She doesn't care if you're possessive, defensive, or lazy—she just wants you to be happy. Happy, happy, happy! This is the kind of world that Venus wants everyone to live in.

In addition to being ruled by Venus, Taurus is a fixed sign. Along with Virgo and Capricorn, it is also one of the earth signs. The earth element gives you your practical nature, and a real dependence upon the comforts of the material world. The fixed quality gives you rigidity, which can make you strong enough to move a mountain but also too inflexible to move it any way but your own. When the earth element and the fixed quality are combined with the happy, harmonizing energies of Venus, true Taurus characteristics emerge. If you express these characteristics in a positive manner you can be strong-willed, warmhearted, sensual, placid, and dependable. Express these characteristics negatively and you can be inflexible, jealous, self-indulgent, bad-tempered, and much too conservative. You need to cultivate your positive characteristics, since your image problem is caused by the infrequent yet unforgettable manifestation of those negative qualities. It hurts you when you behave badly because you are so soft on the inside. You crave harmony and beauty, and you just want everyone to be happy. So isn't it time that you let the whole world know it? Stop giving people the wrong impression of what you're all about. Start dressing like a Taurus, and no one will be confused. You can let everyone know exactly who you are.

YOUR KEYWORD

The keyword *comfortable* needs to be on the mind of every Taurus woman when she is putting together her wardrobe. You have an earthy nature that can be compared to an idyllic green pasture where nothing ever seems to happen. But major disruptions can occur, and when they do they can be catastrophic. It makes no difference whether it's a flood, a drought, or even a tornado touching down, because the pasture cannot fight back. But it can keep growing, and perhaps someday it can reclaim its once-idyllic beauty. You, like this pasture, don't handle disruption well. Nothing bothers you more than being blown out of your comfort zone. But the world of fashion is just as changeable as the weather. Like a bad rainstorm, styles come in and go out overnight. Your challenge is to adapt to the changing circumstances whenever a new fashion climate drifts your way. Once you accept that these changes are inevitable, you can begin to cultivate your own comfortable Taurus style.

YOUR THREE RULES TO DRESS BY

1: Update

Once you get stuck in a rut, it's nearly impossible for you to get out of it. But if you aspire to be cosmically chic, you will have to abandon your comfort zone occasionally to update your wardrobe. Unfortunately, getting yourself to do this can be quite a chore. Your earthy practicality can make you hang on to garments as long as they are functional. Your fixed nature can keep you from adapting when styles have changed. In conjunction, these two forces could make you one of the worst-dressed girls in the zodiac. But you can thank the heavens that Venus is on your side. Venus grants you a highly developed aesthetic sense. You have good taste, Taurus, and you should be able to recognize when something is passé. So don't just sit there while the world of fashion walks on by. Let everyone know how good your taste is by keeping yourself looking up-to-date.

2: Feel Good

Taureans are the most tactile of the zodiac signs. Your earthy sensuality endows you with a well-developed sense of touch. As such, Taurus women rarely purchase clothes that they don't feel good in. Many people can sacrifice a little comfort for a good fit, but not you. Rigid jeans, stiff collars, or tight sweaters do not allow you to feel as comfortable as you want to. If you own items that are restrictive of movement, chances are you barely ever wear them. So don't waste your money. Instead, always buy clothing that appeals to your tactile nature. Soft knitwear, buttery leather, well-worn denim—it doesn't matter what you wear, as long as you love to feel it next to your body. Even if you have to pay a little extra for a particularly comfortable garment, it will be worth it in the long run. Just think of how much you wear the clothes you feel comfortable in. So don't be afraid to open your wallet when comfort is at stake. After all, a cashmere sweater is a cashmere sweater, and cashmere is going to make you feel good.

3: Indulge Wisely

You need to understand that spending money on fashion is an indulgence that you must make in order to look your best. But

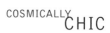
you also ought to realize that opening your wallet is not the only type of indulgence that gives you trouble. Overindulgence can be a problem for you, Taurus. Maybe you eat too much, or smoke too much. Or worse, maybe you shop too much. This can be bad for you, because often women of your sign who overindulge in fashion do it without ever knowing what their personal style is. They buy themselves closets full of fashionable clothes, yet they have no actual style to call their own. You can avoid this problem by putting more thought into what your look is before you purchase anything. It takes more than a fashionable label to make you look great. Learn to indulge wisely, and don't worry about what anyone else is wearing. Just try to look your best in your own signature Taurus style.

SPECIFICS: WHAT TO WEAR

✧ There is a casual, comfortable elegance about a well-dressed Taurus woman. You have an earthy warmth that can put those around you at ease. As such, the colors that you wear well are easy on the eyes. Sandy earth tones and warm, light browns are your best color choices. Soft blues and pale pinks also suit you well.

✧ Blue jeans are definitely a Taurus look. Just don't make them your uniform.

✧ It is likely that you don't wear a lot of bright colors, but for you that can be a good thing. You don't like to clash, even if it's just with the furniture.

✧ Look in your closet. Is everything the same color? That's called a rut.

✧ Most patterns and prints don't do anything for you. However, you could have a fondness for stylized logo patterns, like the double G Gucci designs.

✧ Textured fabrics with interesting patterns woven or knit into them appeal to your tactile nature. It is also likely that you shun synthetic fabrics in favor of natural fibers, such as cotton, linen, or silk.

✧ You love to feel good in your clothes, so knitwear could be your style of choice. In fact, you may indulge in knitwear until your wardrobe becomes very one-dimensional. If that is the case, you should try something else. Knitwear often lacks structure, and it can go only so far in a full wardrobe. The structure and form of woven fabrics and tailored clothing are essential elements in anyone's closet.

✧ You wear tweed well, just as long as the cut of the garment is not too manly.

✧ Many Taurus women are fond of leather, especially in warm, brown shades. A little leather or suede can help you add some diversity to your wardrobe.

✧ If you're the kind of person who wears fur, indulge yourself. The tactility of fur can be irresistible to Taurus women.

✧ One word of caution: Always be sure that you are dressed appropriately for the occasion, since the styles and fabrics you prefer to wear are rather informal.

✧ Many styles work well for you. You may recall those

Ralph Lauren magazine ads from the 1980s in which the models look as if they were just out riding horseback across the English countryside. That is a quintessential Taurus look. However, you can get away with many other styles, as long as they are compatible with your casual, earthy nature.

✧ Since Venus gives you an appreciation for harmony, it is likely that you can mix and match clothes well. Many Taurus women like to wear layered clothing, especially if the layers help you conceal the results of your characteristic overindulgences.

✧ If you prefer skirts to pants, make sure they are not too short. You carry yourself in a fairly relaxed manner, and very short skirts can be a big mistake when you're lounging in a chair, or when you're draped across the sofa in typical Taurus fashion.

✧ You may prefer pants, but only when they are not especially dressy or restrictive of your movement. You detest feeling tied down, whether it's by a man or a pair of tight pants.

✧ Unless you've got money to burn, you usually don't wear dry-clean-only garments when you have an alternative. You hate the menial chore of doing your laundry, but you prefer it to blowing a lot of money on dry-cleaning bills. This is because you are possessive, and when you spend your money you like to have something more than a receipt to show for it.

✧ Looking good requires constant maintenance, Taurus. Even if you don't always feel like putting in the effort that looking your best can require, do yourself a favor and don't let yourself go.

✧ Taurus not only is a feminine sign, but also is ruled by Venus, the most feminine planet. The combined influence of these factors endows Taurus women with a very womanly nature. Taurus women are usually deliriously happy to dress like women.

✧ Although you are normally quite conservative, some of you Taurus women love to play up your sexuality. Looking attractive to the opposite sex is exceptionally enjoyable for you. You may even be the sign that has the most talent for dressing seductively, because your inherent conservativeness can keep you from stepping too far over the line where sexy ends and sleazy begins. But remember that there is a time and a place for every kind of look. So if you are going to dress in a seductive style, make sure you do it in an appropriate manner, and at an appropriate time.

WHO TO WEAR

Ralph Lauren is the designer for you, Taurus. He creates sumptuous, decadent clothing that immediately appeals to your nature. He uses luxurious materials that are wonderful to touch, and his color palette is often heavy on the earth tones. While his designs can be terribly expensive, they are rarely trendy. This is good for you, because when you are comfortable in something you'll want to keep it forever. Paying more for clothes that you know you can wear for a long time isn't a big sacrifice for you. Lauren also designs a few lines, one of which likely falls into your price range. His collections are also knocked off regularly by many of the better department stores' house labels. There is a timeless elegance to his clothing that appeals to the sort of woman who wants to look and feel beautiful without creating waves. You, Taurus, are essentially the most placid creature in the zodiac, and you rarely make waves. That is why the look of Ralph Lauren was made for you.

Another line that suits your Taurean sensibilities is Banana Republic. Their contemporary reinterpretations of classic looks owe a nod of acknowledgment to the style of dressing Ralph Lauren made popular. More often than not, their garments have an earthy feel. Much of their clothing is made with natural fibers, making them even more appealing to you. One-stop shopping in a store like Banana Republic may be all that a Taurus woman like you needs to build up a good, diverse wardrobe. The Gap also suits your sense of style well, providing you with inexpensive casual wear that screams out "comfort zone." You're lucky to have so many choices, Taurus. Just don't get lazy and not bother to make a choice at all.

WHAT TO AVOID

There are two basic types of badly dressed Taurus women. The first type, of course, is the lazy one. She exemplifies the worst of what fashion has to offer by putting no effort into looking good. Maybe she wears poly-cotton knit sweatshirts decorated with kitty-cat faces. Or perhaps she prefers old Birkenstocks and dungarees. It doesn't matter whether she is attractive or not—she looks awful because her clothes look awful. Dressing badly is like having bad manners: Everyone notices you for all the wrong reasons. Just like good manners, fashion sense must be learned. If you don't have any idea what is in style, then you need to learn. Go out and buy yourself some fashion magazines, or beg a store clerk for some help. Better yet, find a well-dressed friend to take you shopping. Just do it, Taurus, and for your own sake do it soon.

The second type of badly dressed Taurus woman is the clotheshorse. She is typically self-indulgent, like most Taureans are, but her self-indulgent tendencies are focused on fashion. She buys and buys whatever catches her eye. She spends too much on items that she believes give her status and style without realizing that style isn't bought—it's created. Instead of combining the items that she has in creative, stylish ways, she fills the holes in her wardrobe by filling the hangers in her closet. If you are one of these Taurus women, you need to stop thinking that spending your money is all it takes to cultivate a sense of style. Put a little more thought into who you are and what you want people to think of you when they see how you are dressed. As well, remember that if anyone is calling you a clotheshorse, you really shouldn't be taking it as a compliment.

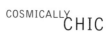
HAIR AND MAKEUP

Each sign reigns over a particular region of the anatomy. For Taurus that area is the mouth and neck. Taurus also rules the vocal cords. Some astrologers claim that Taurus women have beautiful, melodious voices. While that may be true of some of you, there is a more common trait Taureans generally share: You like to talk. You are the zodiac's biggest blabbermouths. So make sure your mouth looks good, since you tend to draw a lot of attention to it. Your lips always must be taken care of. Lip color is an essential element of Taurus style, but don't forget that your lip color needs to be maintained throughout the day. Also, when you visit a cosmetics counter have a clerk assist you in picking out colors, because the wrong shade will not go unnoticed on your noticeable mouth. For the most part your makeup palette is earthy, but a touch of soft blue or pink can go a long way in helping you to liven up your look. As far as the rest of your makeup is concerned, update your cosmetics frequently to avoid getting into a rut or being left behind by fashion. Also please recognize—regardless of how lazy you might feel—that going to bed with your makeup on is a mistake no one ever has to make.

A good hair-care regimen is something that all Taurus women need to develop. Again, laziness is your enemy, and not falling into a rut is your challenge. So make regular appointments with a reputable stylist. Pick a particular day each month, and leave the work to someone else. Most

Taurus women have no preference whether their hair is long or short, but many wear it long just because they cannot bother to get it cut. If this scenario sounds familiar to you, then you should learn to style your hair more creatively. Even simple hair ties or clips can do wonders for you. You should also learn to braid if you have long hair. Many Taureans find the texture of braided hair appealing. However, one of the best things you can do to help your hairstyle is liven it up with a rich, warm color. Taurus women look great with dark blond or medium brown hair and with warm golden highlights. Jet black and platinum blond don't suit your earthy nature at all, and fake colors can make you look simply horrific.

ACCESSORIES

As mentioned before, Taurus rules the neck. Drawing attention to your neck with accessories can help you develop some true Taurus style. Jewelry, especially choker-style necklaces, can ornament and enhance a nice, long neck. Just think of how lovely Audrey Hepburn looked in a simple string of pearls. She was a Taurus. Amber and tortoiseshell accessories can help you dress up your Taurus look, and a gorgeous Hermès scarf is the quintessential Taurus accessory. Scarves are another accessory that Taurus women can have success with. You can become especially sensitive about the way the body part ruled by your sign looks. If this is the case with your neck, scarves can help you conceal that sensitive area. After all, fashion is just as much about concealing what you don't like as it is about showing off what you do like.

Many women have a passion for shoes. You like to go barefoot in your shoes. Never mind how inappropriate it is not to wear the proper hosiery, you can wear out your shoes much faster going barefoot. You, Taurus, just have a thing about comfortable shoes. In fact, you might wear the shoes you like until they fall to pieces. Not even supermodels look good in grungy clothes, so what on earth are you thinking? Keep up your wardrobe, please. Your purse may suffer from the same fate. Next time you buy a purse, remember that in most cases you get what you pay for. If you can spend so much for a shirt that you wear every second week, why not spend a little more on something you carry every day? Indulge yourself, Taurus, and you'll be glad you did. A decadent Fendi bag in the classic two-tone brown color scheme can make you proud to carry a purse, and it matches two colors of shoes. Does life get any better than that?

SOME ADDITIONAL TIPS TO HELP YOU CREATE YOUR OWN COSMIC STYLE

✧ Brush and floss. Dental hygiene is twice as important for someone who always has her mouth open.

✧ A revealing neckline is a must for the Taurus bride. Carry a bouquet of pink gerbera daisies. If you're getting married for the second time, try wearing pink. White wasn't very lucky for you anyway.

✧ Wear earthy, green scents with just a hint of fruit or floral.

✧ Pink or blue flannel pajamas suit your tactile Taurus style. Undergarments in the same colors will appeal to you, too.

✧ Although you can get away with sexy lingerie, it is likely that you prefer simple cotton underwear to lacy bras and frilly panties.

✧ You should avoid very high heels. Your sense of balance isn't all that great, and you can be exceptionally clumsy.

✧ Glen plaids and checks in earthy tones will appeal to you more than most patterns.

✧ Self-maintenance isn't exactly your strong suit. So when you wear nail polish, be sure that you don't let it all chip off before you take the time to redo it.

✧ Remember that "Casual Friday" does not mean "No Socks Friday."

✧ Beige can be your black.

✧ Typical Taurus self-indulgences—smoking, overeating, drinking too much—are not among the secrets to looking good.

✧ If you can get away with a two-piece swimsuit, go for it. Don't forget how sexy Taurus women can be.

A FEW WOMEN WHO — FOR BETTER OR WORSE — EXEMPLIFY TRUE TAURUS STYLE

Barbra Streisand: April 24

With a funky glen plaid hat and honey-blond streaks in her hair, Barbra Steisand has never been sexier than she was in 1972's *What's Up Doc?* Her secret weapon, however, was a tight cardigan sweater that made Babs the babe every Taurus woman yearns to be.

Ann-Margret: April 28

Most Taurus women don't have any idea of how desirable they are. In 1964's *Viva Las Vegas* men were running each other off the road to get next to Ann-Margret in her sexy skirts and pink dresses. With her girl-next-door act she was the epitome of 1960s Taurus chic.

Audrey Hepburn: May 4

Audrey Hepburn is Hollywood's biggest fashion icon. Costumed in her films by the world's top designers, she looked sophisticated and elegant in a way celebrities still try to imitate. Out of character, however, she was a typical Taurean, appearing in interviews dressed in a casual, comfortable style.

Janet Jackson: May 16

Miss Jackson has kind of a nasty way with fashion. It's not that she doesn't wear great clothes but rather that she lets her clothes wear her. Janet Jackson epitomizes the Taurus clotheshorse personality. She would do herself a favor by sticking with the earthy, urban look she wore in her video for 1997's "Got Til It's Gone."

Cher: May 20

Poor Cher! Off-camera she has a laid-back, very Taurean sense of style, which suits her perfectly. But how can anyone forget her on-camera antics? Her self-indulgence has made her the laughingstock of the fashion press. At least performers, though, have an excuse to dress the way they do. After all, they are trying to be remembered, and who could ever forget Cher?

GEMINI
THE TWINS

May 22–June 21

WHAT MAKES YOU
A GEMINI

Gemini, you're a lucky girl. If fashion had a sign of its own, it would be a Gemini. That's because fashion is all about communication, and Geminis were born to communicate. Fashion is about telling people who you are without having to open your mouth. It's a completely effective form of nonverbal communication, just like when you give someone a look that lets him know exactly how you're feeling. Geminis thrive on letting others know how you feel. In fact, making your thoughts and feelings known—instead of keeping things to yourself—is rather healthy for you. You can say anything you want to with your clothing. For you, Gemini, fashion is the universal language that allows you to speak to the world.

Mercury is the ruling planet of your sign. In Roman mythology Mercury was the messenger to the gods. The planet has a similar role in astrology, ruling over the nerves that transmit sensory information to your brain. Mercury enhances your ability to process sensory input, and it improves your ability to communicate that information to others. However, having Mercury as your ruling planet does have a downside. In mythology Mercury was merely a messenger, much like a passenger pigeon with a message tied to its foot. He probably didn't understand much more than the pigeon, either. But he was reliable, quickly getting the message from point A to point B without difficulty. You also communicate both quickly and efficiently, but all too often your understanding of what you're trying to relate is superficial at best. Your mind is quick, but in your haste to communicate you tend to gloss over the details. That's because Mercury has given a rather superficial nature to all those mortals who are born under his favorite sign. Look on the bright side, Gemini: The world of fashion can be superficial, too.

There is much more to what makes you a Gemini than your ruling planet. Gemini is a mutable sign. Being born under a mutable sign makes you adaptable to whatever fate and fortune bring your way. Unfortunately, that same quality can make you a bit unstable. Gemini is also one of the air signs, along with Libra and Aquarius. Individuals born under the air element are the thinkers of the zodiac. When the intellectual orientation of an air sign is combined with the adaptability of a mutable sign, the qualities that make you a Gemini take form. As a result you can be quite versatile, curious, youthful, witty, and communicative. But you also can be inconsistent, superficial, immature, nervous, and two-faced. All of these qualities are part of your personality, Gemini. It's up to you to decide which you would prefer to be remembered for. If you choose the former list, then dressing like a Gemini will only help you enhance those positive qualities. This can be so easy for you, because fickle fashion is always going to be on your side.

YOUR KEYWORD

Duality is your keyword, Gemini, and by recognizing the duality of your air sign you may understand yourself better. Without the oxygen in the air you're breathing, you would quickly perish. But the same air that gives you life is filled with compounds that are harming you at this very moment. Carbon monoxide, radon gas, and many other dangerous chemicals are indistinguishable from the part of the air that allows you to live. Like the different components of the air, the good and bad qualities of a Gemini woman are practically inseparable from one another because they are virtually indistinguishable. What this means, Gemini, is that you must accept that both good and bad things make you who you are.

Once you recognize that duality is in your nature, you will know that dressing in one style all the time is not your style— so don't do it. Instead, dress to please both sides of your nature. The thrill you'll get from looking stylish can be as invigorating to you as a breath of fresh air.

YOUR THREE RULES TO DRESS BY

1: Think

A Gemini woman's mind is much like a machine working in perpetual motion. She never stops thinking of what could happen if events turned out a certain way. When things don't happen in the manner she expects them to, she simply moves on, inventing new scenarios and trying to anticipate what will happen next. She also tells everyone what she's thinking. This is because a Gemini woman finds communication therapeutic, even though what she's saying seems to change from minute to minute. Fashion behaves in a similar manner: It incessantly changes its message to adapt to the many influences that come its way. If you learn to accept that fashion is as fickle as you are, you will be able to think of your adaptability as an advantage. Think about what you want to say with your outfit every time you get dressed. You are the sign of external communication, so think about communicating with every tool you have at your disposal, including your wardrobe. Don't just slap together garments because they match; think about that all-important first impression.

2: Embrace Change

Some signs are very threatened by change, but not you, Gemini. While members of other signs may choose classic looks they can wear for many seasons, you can wear almost anything fashion throws your way. Your adaptability to changing trends is your biggest strength when it comes to putting together a wardrobe. But for a few of you adaptability can seem like a double-edged sword. Maybe you like change too much, in a way that your wallet cannot support. Or maybe you change your look so often that you have no real identity outside the current trend. For you, the key to being cosmically chic is not only to embrace change but also to accept the fact that you are the only sign that moves forward faster than fashion itself. Getting ahead of yourself can make you look like a fool, so don't forget rule 1: Think first; then you can embrace change appropriately.

3: Act Your Age

Mercury gives the members of your sign a youthfulness that other signs just don't have. You were born with a wide-eyed curiosity and a contagious enthusiasm that make you seem eternally young. This youthful outlook also can affect your appearance, keeping you looking and feeling fresh while those around you seethe with envy. Looking young thrills you, but you might find that you play up your youthfulness a bit too much. After all, time waits for no one—not even a young, lively Gemini. So don't get caught wearing tube tops or short-shorts when your age says that your tube-top years are far behind you. You might be saying to yourself, "But age is just a number!" Yes, it is a number, but so is your dress size. The fact that you wore a size four when you were a teenager doesn't necessarily mean you can wear one now. Always be sure to consider those numbers when you are getting dressed.

SPECIFICS: WHAT TO WEAR

- ✧ You're no shrinking violet, Gemini. You are lively, youthful, and exuberant, and you ought to wear colors that will let everyone know what you're all about. Bright yellow, for example, allows you to stand out in a crowd. Not everyone has the skin tone or the hair color to wear yellow successfully, but if anyone belongs in yellow, it's you.

- ✧ Bright blues, hot pinks, vibrant oranges, and the whitest whites also suit you well. Geminis are changeable, and their color palette should reflect that quality. However, you can probably get away with almost any color of the rainbow. Your skin likely has a youthful glow, which is enhanced by wearing bright, saturated colors.

- ✧ A slick yellow raincoat is a look that was made just for you.

- ✧ There are going to be days when you don't feel as mentally sharp or as communicative as you do on others. Tone down the bright colors if doing so makes you feel better, but remember: There are some looks you just don't pull off that well. Dull, monochromatic color schemes or somber tone-on-tone looks are not for you. The same goes for head-to-toe black. You're like the big kid of the zodiac, so don't dress up as if you're a widow in mourning or the daughter of Satan—no one is going to buy it.

✧ Busy patterns suit you well. Many people should avoid complex patterns just to be sure they don't embarrass themselves with a hideous mismatch. Geminis, however, can pull off the most unorthodox combinations of both patterns and garments.

✧ Don't avoid mixing styles just to be on the safe side of fashion. Go ahead and experiment with what you can. There may be trend-setting outfits in your closet that are just waiting to be discovered.

✧ If your youthful charm and naïveté are an excuse for dressing like you're crazy, then why not dress that way? Fashion has a love affair with youth, and teenagers can get away with some pretty crazy looks. This is because naïveté keeps fashion fresh. Eternally youthful Geminis can break all the rules and end up looking incredibly stylish.

✧ The specific garments you wear well always provide you with a lot of freedom of movement. Tight clothes are okay as long as they are stretchy. Short skirts are fine as long as they don't ride up too high. Pants are great, but they must never fit like a plaster cast. Your mind is active, Gemini, and what you wear needs to reflect that fact. If you can move quickly in your clothes, then it is likely that they fit you well.

✧ Many activewear styles appeal to you, as do garments made from light, breezy fabrics. You'll also feel good in shorter dresses—long skirts can make you feel inhibited.

✧ You can be especially fond of athletic clothes and shoes. Just keep in mind that there are places those styles never should go.

✧ You can get away with almost any type of fabric, but you are often more attracted to high-tech synthetics and any other materials that seem new to you.

✧ You should avoid very heavy fabrics, such as velvet, wide-wale corduroy, and thick, wool knits. Don't ever let your outfit weigh you down.

✧ Airy clothes that breathe well appeal to every Gemini woman's comfort zone.

✧ You have the ability to change your mood by adapting your look. For you, Gemini, changing your state of mind can be as easy as changing your outfit.

✧ Your ruling planet can help you to develop some true Gemini chic. Mercury rules over early education. So, schoolgirl looks are a classic Gemini style. While adopting this look whole-heartedly may be inappropriate for most Gemini women, elements of this style can go far for you. For instance, oxford shirts with skinny ties, kneesocks, and even those short tartan skirts seem to come back into fashion every other season. You may have luck with them yourself.

✧ Garments emblazoned with letters, words, or sayings are a typical Mercurial style.

✧ Anything designed with the connotation of travel—especially flight—is appealing to a Gemini woman. When a designer's collection seems to be inspired by a vacation to an exotic land, that inspiration is also a Mercurial influence. You can pick up many great ideas from Mercury. He's never too far from the flighty world of fashion, which he loves.

WHO TO WEAR

Because the idea of fashion has so much in common with your sign, the designer for you would have to be Karl Lagerfeld. He is an embodiment of the spirit of fashion itself. Although he seems to be inspired by the past, he manages to make his designs seem modern—or even futuristic. But regardless of where he derives his inspiration, the collections that spring forth from his imagination rewrite the rules of fashion season after season. His styles communicate the wearer's willingness to adapt her own look in order to dive into the world of fashion headfirst. His ready-to-wear lines for Chanel are made for versatile women who radiate youthfulness and vitality. But don't despair if Chanel is way out of your price range, because many other designers of ready-to-wear fashions copy him ruthlessly. Just use that quick mind of yours, Gemini. First, study the Chanel runway shows. Take note of the styles you would like to re-create. With a little thought and effort you can steal any look that appeals to you. In your own superficial way, you too can be a Chanel woman.

There are many other labels that suit Gemini women well. Lagerfeld's clothes for the Fendi label are funky and trend-setting. Anna Sui is a terrific designer whose youthful creations have an undeniable charm. Max Azria's BCBG line is trendy, fun, and not that expensive. In addition to designer labels, many chain stores can serve you well, offering trendy clothes that are economically priced—usually because they are marketed to teenagers. If you think you can get away with clothes like that, you're probably right—just remember to act your age! Moreover, do yourself a favor and think twice before you spend your money. The return policies at retail stores are rarely as adaptable as you are, and you have been known to change your mind about a purchase before you've even left the mall.

WHAT TO AVOID

The worst-dressed Gemini women are living a lie. They have decided that a certain look defines them perfectly, and that outside that look fashion has nothing to offer them. All of you Geminis must accept that duality is in your nature, and that adaptability is your greatest strength. Otherwise, your wardrobe can begin to seem like a one-line joke—it's just not very funny when you are the punch line. Perhaps you work in a downtown office and have decided that you look great in your power suits. That's no reason to put on an uptight business suit every day of the week. Suppose you really enjoyed the *Flashdance* look of the 1980s. That's no reason to still be wearing leg warmers today. Not only do you need to forget the past but you also must learn to embrace the duality of your sign. Your dual nature can allow you to be any kind of beautiful woman that you want to be. All you need to do is try, Gemini. Don't ever be afraid to be fashionable.

Another problem that many Gemini women have is they can try too hard to make a lasting first impression. While the importance of first impressions has been mentioned, the pitfalls of making a bad first impression must be discussed. Think of your fellow Gemini Cyndi Lauper. Although her career took her in many directions, and through several different styles, that first glimpse of her etched an indelible image into the mind of the public—or at least into the mind of anyone old enough to remember her when she arrived on the pop music scene. Years later she is still remembered for the goofy, antiestablishment style that helped to make her a star. All of you Geminis have the ability to be trendsetters, like Cyndi Lauper, but you also ought to realize that if you define yourself with a characteristic look, you could live to regret it.

HAIR AND MAKEUP

If there was a sign whose members were born to wear short hair, it would have to be yours. Sassy, boyish cuts suit your on-the-go lifestyle. But many women refuse to wear their hair short. Often this is because the men in their lives express a preference for long hair. So think about this, Gemini. If a man appreciates you, he's going to appreciate you with the haircut that makes you feel good. But if long hair is what makes you happy, then be sure to keep your haircut versatile and adaptable to what fashion currently dictates. Don't let a bad-hair day turn into a bad-hair life. At all costs, avoid big hairdos. Color changes also can help you keep your hairdo in fashion. Gemini women often make the best blondes, simply because of the association of fair hair with youth. At least consider becoming a blonde at some point in your life. It may be more fun than you can imagine. Vibrant colors may appeal to you as well. After a couple of good dye jobs you may even find yourself addicted to the process. For you, Gemini, updating your look can be the most rewarding habit.

Your makeup palette must also undergo many changes. Keeping your look fresh and lively means making sure your cosmetics are just as fresh. In addition, you should experiment with new products and application techniques. Chances are you'll be thrilled with the results. For inspiration take a look at what teenagers are doing with their hair and makeup. Just consider your own age when you adapt these styles. Masking wrinkles with heavy makeup doesn't make anyone look younger. Also, try to stay away from dark colors and high-contrast combinations, such as dark lipstick and pale foundation. Looking like a vampire just isn't your style.

ACCESSORIES

Since you are known as the great communicator of the zodiac, you might expect that your sign would rule over speech and the vocal cords. However, the type of communication Gemini is associated with is much broader than speech. Gemini rules the hands and arms. Whether you are dialing a phone, writing a novel, or typing a letter, your hands are an indispensable accessory to your communicative abilities. Therefore, accessorizing your hands is an important element of Gemini style. Start by taking care of your hands. If you don't, people might notice only your chewed nails and ragged cuticles instead of whatever you are trying to say. Nail polish is also essential. You should change your nail color like you change your underwear. Let your fingernails be your jewelry, but exercise some caution when it comes to jewelry itself. Many poorly dressed Gemini women wear way too many rings at the same time. One or two rings make a much more fashionable statement than nine or ten. For the sake of good taste, don't let your fingers look like a scrap heap. Learn to treat your hands like a part of your wardrobe, and you'll find that they can do a lot more for you than just open doors.

Silver jewelry generally appeals to Gemini women more than gold, but that's no reason not to have both—and platinum, too!

The influence of Mercury is important when other accessories are considered. Shoes must allow for swift movement. Your lifestyle is active and you move rather swiftly, so try to buy shoes that have some grip in the soles. Hosiery must fit well and be youthful in design—no old-lady knee-highs for you, Gemini. Colorful socks and hosiery are a great addition to your wardrobe. Don't be afraid of patterned hose either. Your sunglasses, hair hardware, and jewelry are rarely expensive, since you normally prefer a wardrobe of accessories to just a few pricey items. Purses are purchased with the same thought. Unless you're rich, you would probably be better off with a couple of inexpensive, trendy bags every season or two, rather than with one or two costly classics. Suit yourself, Gemini, but always be sure that a new purse has plenty of room for the ultimate Gemini accessory: your cellular phone. For a communicative Gemini woman, a cellular phone is like a security blanket.

SOME ADDITIONAL TIPS TO HELP YOU CREATE YOUR OWN COSMIC STYLE

✧ Fresh scents with a hint of citrus suit a Gemini woman well.

✦ A bright, floral-printed swimsuit can make you a show-off at the beach.

✦ Even though a short skirt may seem untraditional for a bridal dress, it is the perfect length for you. Carry a bouquet of fragrant white flowers down the aisle, such as freesia or orange blossoms.

✦ Keeping those hands of yours young-looking is a must. Always carry hand lotion in your purse.

✦ Sexy baby-doll pajamas can heat up your bedroom all winter long.

✦ Bras and panties in lightweight, stretchy fabrics will suit you better than heavy support garments and clunky underwires.

✦ Because Gemini rules over the arms, you could be sensitive about the way your arms look. Do yourself a favor, Gemini—stop whining and get to the gym.

✦ Remember that "Casual Friday" does not mean "Tank-Top Friday." The office rarely is the place for bare armpits.

A FEW WOMEN WHO— FOR BETTER OR WORSE— EXEMPLIFY TRUE GEMINI STYLE

Stevie Nicks: May 26

This songbird's style is as tired now as it was in the 1970s. Incapable of embracing change, Stevie Nicks doesn't even

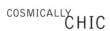
come close to dressing up to the potential of her Gemini sun sign. In her same-old, same-old gypsy attire, she's a role model for bag ladies everywhere.

LaToya Jackson: May 29

Geminis are supposed to be the great communicators of the zodiac, but somehow Michael and Janet's sister just seems to say the same three words over and over again: "I'm a mess . . . I'm a mess . . . I'm a mess."

Brooke Shields: May 31

While many other child performers have outgrown their looks, Brooke Shields has managed to maintain the youthful glow that helped make her a star. She will always be a Pretty Baby. Dressed in trendy, active looks, she belies her age beautifully in typical Gemini style.

Marilyn Monroe: June 1

With her breezy white dress and butter-blond hair, Marilyn Monroe gave us one of cinema's most memorable moments in *The Seven Year Itch* (1955). But even though that look was pure, perfect Gemini style, it was Marilyn's youthful vitality—a Gemini woman's best quality—that made the scene a classic.

Steffi Graf: June 14

The association between swift movement and the sign of Gemini is demonstrated ideally in the quickness of Steffi Graf. On the tennis court she always looks great in those short, sporty skirts, just as a Gemini should.

CANCER
THE CRAB

June 22–July 22

WHAT MAKES YOU
A CANCER

Nobody really wants to be a Cancer. Not only does your sign share its name with a dread disease but you also have the misfortune of being represented by the worst symbol in the zodiac: the crab. Having such a lousy symbol wouldn't be all that bad if you were the most upbeat girl in the zodiac— but you're not. In fact, you can be quite crabby. However, just as often you can be easygoing, or sullen, or cheerful, or nervous, or any other mood imaginable. This is because profound mood swings are the hallmark of your sign, and everyone knows it. It's likely that the people around you tread quite lightly, because they want to know what kind of mood you're in before they say or do the wrong thing. You can be so touchy sometimes that you may wonder why anyone bothers to come around you at all. But they do, and the reason why is this: You have a good side. As a matter of fact, you can be the sweetest crab anyone has ever met. Your good side is so good that everyone has learned to love you despite your bad side. You should be glad to know this, Cancer, because if there is one thing that can change your mood from bad to good, it is to feel loved and wanted by the people you love yourself.

Cancer is ruled by the moon. While the planets can take months—or even years—to move through a single sign of the zodiac, the moon speeds through each sign every couple of days. With each move, the moon touches a different nerve in you, changing your moods, altering your perspectives, and reordering your priorities. The phase of the moon also affects you profoundly, and eclipses can change your personality for better or worse. But the moon endows you with more than just a moody nature. In mythology the moon ruled over the principle of motherhood. Consequently, most Cancers have a rather intense need to love and nurture the people around you. However, you also may find yourself acting upon some less desirable motherly impulses. For instance, you can smother people with affection, overwhelming them with your protective nature. You also can be exceptionally needy. Yet no one is going to tell you that, because you will inevitably fight back with the one weapon that all Cancers were born to use: guilt. The maternal influence of the moon has given you the ability to make people feel sorry for you. Nevertheless, you shouldn't let this one characteristic become a predominant aspect of your personality, or your overt neediness could drive everyone away from you—and that's not at all what you want.

Along with Scorpio and Pisces, Cancer is one of the water signs. Individuals born under a water sign feel their way through the world. Emotional gratification is more important to them than anything else. Cancer is also a cardinal sign. People who are born under a cardinal sign have a linear thought process and a pragmatic character. The steadying influence of the cardinal quality keeps most Cancers from becoming complete emotional wrecks. When the focused nature of the cardinal quality is blended with the sensate nature of the water element, the characteristics that make you a Cancer become apparent. On the positive side you can be sensitive, intuitive, nurturing, tenacious, and remarkably creative. On the negative side you can be moody, oversensitive, overprotective, worrisome, and—contrary to your cardinal nature—fearful of the future. You can emphasize your positive side by recognizing that your feelings are not completely under the control of external forces, such as the moon. You must develop a strong sense of security about yourself that will allow others to see your good side regardless of your frame of mind. By dressing impeccably you can give people the impression that you are in control of yourself. Your wardrobe

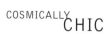

can be a tough crab shell that protects your soft insides from whatever the cruel world brings your way.

YOUR KEYWORD

Think of the water that symbolizes your sign as a pond in a subterranean cave. Not only is the pond protected by the rocky walls surrounding it but it is also fed by an underground spring that keeps it fresh and full of life. Inside the pond are fish who have evolved depending upon the safety of this environment. To them this pond is like a mother, for without it they would not exist. The fish have lived in the pond for countless generations, and with the cave walls to protect them there is no reason to believe that this placid scenario will ever come to an end. In a word, this environment is secure. For a Cancer woman, security is probably the most important issue in your life. In fact, *security* is your keyword, Cancer. Like the fish in the pond, you thrive on knowing that you can depend on the stability of your surroundings. Therefore, security ought to play an important part in the way you dress. Think of your wardrobe as the rock walls that will protect the delicate environment under your skin. If you appear to be secure on the outside, no one will ever have to know how fragile you can be on the inside. For you, Cancer, being well-dressed and feeling secure about yourself go hand in hand.

YOUR THREE RULES TO DRESS BY

1: Dress Defensively

Because emotional security plays a crucial role in your success, you must approach putting together a wardrobe with a rather defensive attitude. You need to look so secure on the outside that no one will ever have to question what's going on inside that head of yours. The secret to building up the kind of wardrobe that will defend your vulnerable psyche is this: Dress in a style that makes people take you seriously. Find garments that were designed to be worn for years, and avoid trends whenever you can. Although following this advice may not make you seem especially fashionable, it will definitely make you seem more credible. For example, think of the type of clothing that people with "old money" wear. Do you remember seeing John F. Kennedy, Jr., or his wife, Carolyn, looking terribly trendy? Of course not. But they did look credible, and they always looked great. That's because being rich never goes out of fashion, and neither does looking rich. Adopting a similar style can help you look and feel secure even when you're in one of your dreariest, most vulnerable moods. By dressing defensively in a universally appealing style you'll just feel better.

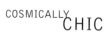
2: Don't Look Back

People who are born under a cardinal sign generally have a forward-looking disposition. But being ruled by the moon makes Cancers quite fond of the past. You look back on history with rose-colored glasses, and many of you find yourselves feeling nostalgic for a moment in time that you didn't live through. The conflict between your forward-looking cardinal nature and the backward-looking nature of the moon can make it difficult for you to define yourself with a particular style. But you ought to forget the past and embrace the present. Contemporary classics suit you much better than secondhand bargains. This is because your sense of the past is often idealized. You can embarrass yourself by attempting to resurrect styles that are not ready to come back. Try to build up a wardrobe that is modern and fashion-forward, and leave the retro looks to those who have a genuine feeling for the past, not just a fondness for it. Only then will you find the security that you thrive on.

3: Be Positive

A Cancer woman's insecurity about her looks can be quite tragic. Even the most beautiful Cancer women are especially hard on themselves. You are so sensitive that you can become depressed by misinterpreting a harmless comment or a passing glance. You've got to adopt a more positive attitude about yourself. Don't fret if your mirror shows every imperfection on your body, because it also shows all the good parts. When you really know yourself, you can use fashion to accentuate the positive elements of your look, and you can learn to downplay those things you don't like about yourself. Make a conscious effort to accentuate the positive, Cancer, and you'll look and feel better. Nothing makes a beautiful face look worse than a frown, so cheer up! Always look to the bright side of things and you'll discover that beauty really does come from within.

SPECIFICS: WHAT TO WEAR

✧ If there was one safe color for anyone to wear, that color would have to be black. Consequently, many Cancer women find a sense of security by wearing black on a regular basis.

✧ While it is difficult to go wrong with black, you ought to be aware that wearing dark colors too often can be a mistake. Every Cancer woman should lighten up her color palette. The entire blue spectrum is ideal for you. Silver, gray, white, and soft lavender also will go a long way in adding variety to your wardrobe.

✧ Striking a balance between the dark and light colors you wear is an ideal way to look more approachable. Wearing head-to-toe dark colors can be rather intimidating. For someone who thrives on feeling loved and wanted, making others feel intimidated by your appearance is a recipe for disaster. Don't avoid dark colors altogether. Just don't let them become your uniform.

✧ Learn to dress appropriately for the season. For many poorly dressed Cancer women it can seem like winter all year long.

✧ All women born under a water sign can benefit from utilizing fluid fabrics in their wardrobes. The stiffness of a boxy blazer, for instance, can be tempered by a fluid, less-structured blouse, or an elegant, soft knit top. Combining hard and soft layers should come naturally to a woman who is—like the crab she is symbolized by—the perfect combination of hard and soft qualities.

✧ Chunky knitwear is definitely not for you, but smaller-scale knits can give your wardrobe a boost. Try wearing more jersey, for example.

✧ Fabrics with a slightly reflective surface, like sharkskin, might find their way into your closet. Dresses made of satiny fabrics look great on Cancer women, too. So do sheer fabrics and meshlike knits. Avoid very loose-fitting clothing because you shouldn't try to disguise your figure.

✧ Suede can be a good choice for you as well, but you should avoid wearing too much leather. Black leather has an edginess that can make a Cancer woman look rather unapproachable. Save the leather for your shoes and purses, and you won't have to worry about scaring people away with a look that's just not your style.

✧ It is likely that structured, tailored garments appeal to you. Suits, in particular, are an ideal choice for a Cancer woman. Just be careful that you don't wear this hard-edged style of clothing exclusively.

- ✦ Cancers generally let their nostalgia affect the way they express themselves through fashion. A preference for either skirts or pants is present in most Cancer women, and their choice is often based on which garments they wore more comfortably as a child.
- ✦ You often wear clothing that fits close to your body. Cancer is a feminine sign, and possessing a feminine shape is important to most Cancer women. Well-defined hips and an obvious waistline are essential, but more often you emphasize your top half most deliberately. The reason for this is that your sign rules over the breasts, and having a shapely bustline is of paramount importance to you. When current styles allow for it, try to wear more body-hugging tops.
- ✦ You probably get a thrill out of dresses and jackets that flatter your most prized possessions. Sweaters and shirts are often chosen for how they accentuate your bust, and many of you enjoy revealing a little cleavage. However, try not to go overboard showing off your bosom. Too many badly dressed Cancer women dive into the world of fashion chest-first. There is a difference between sexy and tacky. Please learn to distinguish between the two.
- ✦ Prints and patterns can help you make your wardrobe more interesting. The moon, your ruling planet, rules over plants and flowers. A floral print can be quite pretty on you, and it can give your look a soft edge that others will find appealing.

✧ Be careful to choose prints and patterns that are not too garish. Simple pinstripes, especially in silvery grays, are a good choice for you. In fact, a pin-striped navy suit is the quintessential Cancer garment. If you don't own one now, make purchasing one a priority.

WHO TO WEAR

No other designer makes clothing that suits a Cancer woman better than Giorgio Armani. Season after season Armani devotees depend upon the Italian designer to produce another completely wear- 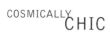 able collection, and he never disappoints his fans. By creating classical, elegant clothing with an emphasis on luxurious fabrics, Armani has built a fashion empire that is envied worldwide. Celebrities, politicians, and even royalty are among his clients. The reason these people wear Armani is they know they will look great regardless of the current trends. Armani is better than any other designer at bridging the gap between that "old money" look and contemporary style. Armani is surely the world's safest label to wear, and for that reason alone it is the ideal choice for all security-loving Cancer women. And for those of you who love financial security, don't despair if the Armani signature labels are way out of your price range, because A/X Armani Exchange offers hip, less-expensive clothes that suit your Cancer style perfectly.

There are many other "safe" labels a Cancer woman can

have success with. For instance, St. John by Marie Gray is about as safe as safe gets. As well, many in-house labels at finer department stores are a good choice for you. This is because department store lines are generally understated and not terribly trendy. Still, some Cancer women like to take a walk on the wild side every now and then, in something like a Hervé Leger dress. Leger designed those sexy, elastic-fabric numbers that every supermodel and celebrity with a nice body wore in the 1980s. His signature garment was a tight, short dress that fit like a girdle, defining every bump and curve. If you've got a nice figure, Cancer, don't be afraid to wear your clothing skintight. You were born to wear your clothes as tight as a crab shell. It's in the stars.

WHAT TO AVOID

The most common mistake Cancer women make is wearing dark colors too often. Choosing too many severely tailored garments also can be a problem, and many badly dressed Cancer women find themselves looking quite uptight. But the worst mistake you can make is sporting clothes that are best described as matronly. You sometimes wear somber, boring outfits that add years to your appearance. If this scenario sounds familiar, you've got to snap out of it, Cancer! When given the chance to look better or worse, why on earth would you choose worse? By trying to make yourself look nondescript, you look awful in your uninteresting, unfashionable attire.

For example, think of your fellow Cancer Princess Diana. When she married Prince Charles, she tried to fit into her new family by adopting the matronly style of the Windsor women. Criticizing her lack of personal style became a sport for fashion know-it-alls everywhere. But instead of retreating from the criticism—like many other Cancers would have done—Diana enlisted the aid of designers worldwide. Without taking any chances with trendy clothes, she was able to transform herself into one of the world's most fashionable women. By wearing elegant, modern styles, and abandoning the stuffy tradition of her in-laws, Diana became a fashion icon without ever becoming a trendsetter. Every Cancer woman should learn from Diana's mistakes and aspire to make herself more stylish. After all, the whole world may be watching you, too.

HAIR AND MAKEUP

Many Cancer women find themselves wearing a hair color that is far too dark for their skin tone. Regardless of season, any time is the right time for you to lighten up your look. Even a small change in your hair color can work wonders with your appearance. Go a shade lighter, or indulge yourself by getting some natural-looking highlights. Furthermore, don't worry if the years are creeping up on you, because no one makes a better-looking silver fox than a Cancer woman. Just go with the flow! However, be careful to avoid stiff, severe hairstyles. Relaxing a stiff hairdo can help you look and feel more attractive. Likewise, try to avoid tying your hair back whenever possible, because nothing says "uptight" like a bun. More important, learn to go easy on the styling products. Without a doubt, Cancer women are the zodiac's most notorious hair-spray addicts.

The same kind of advice applies to your makeup. First, make sure your foundation isn't too dark for your complexion. Then lighten up your look with a big dose of color. Many shades of blue can go far in your makeup palette. So can frosty silvers and pearly whites. In fact, any product with a hint of pearly sheen is perfect for your Cancer look. Adding a little contour to your face also may appeal to you. Many of you have round, moonlike faces, so adding emphasis to your bone structure is necessary. However, be wary of going over the top when trying to give definition to your features. Learn to work with what you've got, and don't expect miracles. And, by all means, don't let anyone convince you that more makeup equals more beauty. The way you apply your cosmetics needs to be just as light as the colors you should be wearing. And take some precautionary measures when venturing into the daylight. Your skin may be unusually sensitive to the sun.

ACCESSORIES

Because the sign of Cancer rules over the bosom, a Cancer woman needs to treat brassieres as accessories to her wardrobe and not as a necessary evil that accompanies having breasts. A good bra should be something you're glad to wear. First of all, it should fit you well. Clothes hang much better on a woman who is wearing the correct bra size. If your bra is cutting into your back, or if it's not offering you any support, get a new one—it's as simple as that. As well, remember that certain styles can show off your bra, through a sheer fabric or a tightly knit top, and your bra can make or break an outfit. So don't conclude that your bra is not an essential piece of your wardrobe just because it's underneath your clothing. If you put a little more effort into finding yourself the right bra, your entire look will benefit from it.

There are other accessories that you also need to put more effort into finding. Purses, shoes, and belts should be purchased for their classic simplicity, since these items generally last through several seasons. Avoid trendy styles, and try to stick to a limited color scheme. If you are one of the many Cancer women who adores wearing black, this is the one part of your wardrobe where black is the best option. Classic lines like Chanel, Dior, and Gucci are good choices for you. But they are expensive, so be sure to select styles that won't look foolish in a year, and try to purchase coordinating pieces together. Also, wearing hosiery that is too dark is a bad habit you may need to break. It may sound like a cliché, but for the well-dressed Cancer woman the shoes have got to match the bag—and the belt, too.

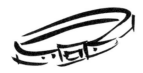

SOME ADDITIONAL TIPS TO HELP YOU CREATE YOUR OWN COSMIC STYLE

✧ You should stick to the classics when wearing perfume.

✧ Pearlized nail polish looks great on you, Cancer. Frosted or shimmery cosmetics also suit you well.

✧ Whenever your outfit is in need of a boost, a good push-up bra will do the trick.

✧ A traditional, elegant wedding dress is pure Cancer style. Carry a bouquet of icy white orchids.

✧ Your self-sacrificing, maternal nature could make you neglect your own needs when you've got kids to take care of. Try your best not to let yourself go.

✧ A one-piece swimsuit in a watery color will appeal to you. You may find a suit with padded cups desirable as well.

✧ Sleepwear in fluid, luxurious fabrics is a must-have for all Cancer women.

✧ If you're stressed out, be sure you're not wearing your anxiety on your face. Worry lines run twice as deep on a Cancer woman's brow.

✧ Remember that "Casual Friday" means it is time to relax and dress down a little. Don't be a stick-in-the-mud and wear the same old things you always wear.

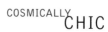
A FEW WOMEN WHO — FOR BETTER OR WORSE — EXEMPLIFY TRUE CANCER STYLE

Princess Diana: July 1

Diana was one of the fashion world's greatest success stories. By taking her inner suffering out into the open, the Princess of Wales attracted the pity of the top designers. In a few years, she was able to go from dowdy to dynamic with a little help from her stylish friends.

Pamela Anderson: July 1

Most Cancer women could benefit from playing up their sexuality more often. The actress Pamela Anderson, however, goes above and beyond what a woman needs to do to make herself more attractive. With her ultrafake femininity, she has reinvented herself into fashion's Bride of Frankenstein.

Nancy Reagan: July 6

The 1980s were defined by a forced glamour that is demonstrated ideally by former First Lady Nancy Reagan. In her severe suits and overwrought evening wear, she was perfectly fashionable for the time. But, in retrospect, she never took any chances with her wardrobe, and her eighties look now seems as unattractively uptight as her demeanor.

Courtney Love: July 9

When she finally dropped her antifashion pose and realized how stylish she could be, the pop star Courtney Love saw herself become the darling of the fashion press. Like a typical Cancer woman, she seems to become more and more beautiful when she knows that she is adored by others.

Diahann Carroll: July 17

The groundbreaking actress Diahann Carroll is simply divine. By carefully choosing her wardrobe pieces, she is able to stay current without sacrificing the classically beautiful look that defines her perfectly. She's a shining example of that "old money" look that suits Cancer women so very well.

CHAPTER FIVE

LEO
THE LION

July 23–August 22

WHAT MAKES YOU A LEO

Leo, you are the queen of the zodiac—or at least you like to think so. In fact, nothing pleases you more than when you are treated like royalty. But rather than being the kind of queen who would throw a pitiful peasant in the dungeon just to prove she could, you wield your power in a far more benevolent manner. This is because you are gracious. Despite your stellar ego, you are probably the most gracious monarch the zodiac has ever known. You're always eager to lend your loyal subjects a helping hand. You will feed them, clothe them, and put roofs over their heads. You'll do whatever they need because you are their beloved queen, Leo. But there is a limit to how benevolent you can be. When impertinent fools venture to ask why it is your word and not theirs that reigns supreme, you do not hesitate to let them know who is in charge. And you have a special way of dealing with the kinds of people who take your generosity for granted. Like the heads of the traitors who have betrayed you, you simply cut them off.

The reason you need to be worshiped like a queen is your ruling planet. Leo is ruled by the sun, the undisputed monarch of our astrological universe. The sun gives your personality a rather magnetic quality, much like a gravitational force that draws others toward you. It is only natural for you to be surrounded by an entourage of heavenly bodies. To this loyal retinue you confer warmth, light, and energy. On the one hand, you are charity personified, selflessly endowing your vitality to those you choose to shine upon. On the other hand, your adversaries are no more important to you than cosmic debris caught up in your gravitational pull. Sure, you may shine on them like you shine on everyone else, but your sunny disposition can't fool them. In time they realize that it is the awesome magnitude of your personality that brightens up their dim lives, not vice versa.

The sun is not alone in determining aspects of your personality. Like Aries and Sagittarius, Leo is a fire sign. It is also one of the fixed signs. The fire element adds intuition and passion to your personality. The fixed quality adds stability and self-assuredness. Combined with the influence of your ruling planet, these factors give rise to typical Leo characteristics. Positive Leo character traits include great willpower, artistic creativity, generosity, vivaciousness, and personal aplomb. However, negative Leo character traits include stubbornness, egotism, self-righteousness, self-indulgence, and an overt theatricality. In astrology the sun represents your sense of self-expression, and it is the primary indicator of how your positive and negative qualities are expressed externally. Fashion is also concerned with external self-expression. For this reason, you should not find it difficult to express yourself with your wardrobe. With very little effort you can create a self-image that allows you to shine more brilliantly than any other sign in the zodiac.

YOUR KEYWORD

Drama is the keyword you must remember when putting together a wardrobe. Your Leo fire is much like the pent-up fire in a dormant volcano. Although a volcano can be majestic and imposing in its dormant state, it is far more exciting when active. A little burst of ash here and there, a puff of smoke now and then, or even the occasional rumble just aren't enough: It's the drama of the eruption that makes everyone stand up and take notice. No one can deny the power of a volcano when it's shaking the earth, spewing fire, and embellishing its slopes with rivers of molten rock. Like this volcano, the well-dressed Leo woman always gives her audience something spectacular to look at. You possess an undeniable amount of power when you are performing, and you must deliver a performance that gets you noticed. Drama will get you the attention that you deserve. Remember, the whole world is expecting you to put on a show. Don't disappoint them. If you choose to be dormant, you'll just blend into the surroundings. But if you choose to be fiery and dramatic, you'll shake the earth that's under their feet.

YOUR THREE RULES TO DRESS BY

1: Define Your Character

Image means everything to the typical Leo woman. So, the public face she presents should be an accurate representation of her powerful, magnetic personality. The best-dressed Leo woman uses her innate sense of creativity to craft a look that defines her personality ideally. By spending money wisely, and avoiding impulse purchases whenever possible, she is able to create a wardrobe that radiates individual character. There is nothing improvisational about the way she appears, yet she never fails to surprise her audience with her fashion choices. The reason she always looks so well-rehearsed is that she truly knows who she is. You, Leo, can be well-dressed simply by knowing yourself inside and out. Think of the world as your stage, and define your own character like a part in a play. If you stick to this script, you'll be sure to deliver an award-winning performance every time you get dressed.

2: Show Off

Most Leo women profess a fondness for dressing up in costumes. You love to express your creativity to the world, and dressing in theatrical costumes allows you to show off your artistic side. However, if you think you've grown out of this childhood phase, perhaps you should think again. You are a born performer, and choosing garments that have dramatic flair is second nature to you. This is because no one else can show off an ensemble with more aplomb than you can. You are the supermodel of the zodiac strutting down the catwalk, dripping with confidence and attitude. So work it for all that it's worth! Dress up to get attention, and don't ever let mediocrity get the best of you. Let your courageous nature and instinctive creativity help you show off a wardrobe that only a proud, showy Leo could get away with. Your own sense of self-assurance is the one thing that can turn a simple outfit into a sight to behold.

3: Dress for Yourself

How you dress is often determined by factors that seem to be beyond your control. For instance, if you work in an office, you are usually required to adhere to a rather austere dress code. Many social occasions also require a style of dressing

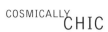
that just doesn't appeal to you. Finding a way to express your own personality within situations like these can be a genuine art form. Fortunately for you, artistic creativity is something that Leos possess in spades. Your artful nature can be the one factor that allows you to make your wardrobe more special than just a closet full of uniforms. You hate uniforms. You abhor being told what to wear just as much as you dislike being told what to do, but your competitive nature rarely allows you to acquiesce so willingly. If you are up to the challenge, you can find a way to individualize any outfit you are required to wear. You simply look better when you dress for yourself, but sometimes you must make a point of playing by the rules. Just don't forget that bending the rules to suit your own needs is something you were born to do. It's in the stars.

SPECIFICS: WHAT TO WEAR

✧ It should come as no surprise to you that Leos look great in bright, sunny colors. But instead of wearing the purest shades of red, yellow, and orange, try to wear colors that appear a little sunburnt. For example, the burnt orange color of a terra-cotta clay pot suits you ideally, and the same can be said about the glorious golden color of a wheat field just before harvest.

✧ Even though the sun enters the sign of Leo in midsummer, the breathtaking colors of autumn leaves can be flattering on you. Burnt sienna suits you, too.

✧ Don't worry if your skin tone does not allow you to wear typical Leo hues, because nothing says drama like a bold combination of colors. For instance, anyone can get away with black and white, but when someone like you dons this most classic combination, the results are stunning rather than classic.

✧ Many other high-contrast color combinations also look great on you. If you are going to make an effort to stand out in the crowd—and you should—dramatic color combinations can be the cornerstone of your wardrobe.

✧ You should try to avoid wearing too many neutral colors, pastels, or gray tones. Your regal presence allows you to command attention regardless of what you're wearing, but that alone is no reason to cultivate a personal style that simply blends into the background.

✧ In general, there are no specific types of garments that complement you better. Skirts or pants, high heels or flats, skintight or baggy—it doesn't make a great deal of difference what you wear, because it is the manner in which you wear your clothes that makes them your own.

✧ You are implicitly creative, and you can build a great outfit with the materials you have on hand. For this reason it is likely that you are the only girl in the zodiac who should stockpile her old clothing. Keep your closet full and keep your options open.

✧ Truly stylish Leos wear what they want regardless of what is supposed to be fashionable. Whether they are sporting the hottest labels or wearing thrift shop bargains, they combine style with attitude in a way that makes them seem like they know fashion better than anyone else.

✧ Madonna is a Leo, and she wears everything she owns with an aplomb that no one else could get away with. Even when she looks outrageous, her personal style still intimidates everyone around her. The cosmos has given all of you Leos the gift of absolute personal style: the ability to dictate what everyone else should be wearing. You will always have the last word on what is in fashion, and you should not be afraid to voice it.

✧ Your personal style benefits greatly by the addition of dramatic pieces to your wardrobe. For instance, a fur coat, whether it's real or fake, can make you feel like a celebrity every time you make your cinematic entrance.

✧ Many exotic animal hides—like snakeskin, lizard, or alligator—may seem as if they were put on this earth just for you to wear. It takes a certain kind of woman to get away with wearing feathers as well, but you are that kind of woman, Leo.

✧ Leopard spots, zebra stripes, and many other outlandish animal prints can add some real drama to your closet.

✧ An ideal way to add some excitement to your look is to wear clothing that has been designed with exaggerated proportions. For instance, a blazer with a nipped waistline and square, padded shoulders will suit you much more than a classically cut jacket. Pants that are very narrow-legged or those adorned with tremendously wide flares will also suit you better than a classic, straight-legged look.

✧ You should do your best to avoid classically cut clothing altogether. Because Leo is a fixed sign, you can be a little suspicious of change, and the reason the classics are called the classics is that they barely ever change. Don't get stuck in that rut, Leo. Spartan classics are never going to make you look like the superstar you know you are.

✧ Having the sun as your ruling planet influences the type of clothing you look best in. Glitzy gold fabrics, such as Lurex or lamé, suit you Leo women well. Most women would have a difficult time wearing such flashy clothes, but not you. Nevertheless, you should try to avoid wearing clothing that is glitzy too often, or you could start to look as if you should be serving cocktails in a Las Vegas casino.

✧ Leo also rules the back, and for this reason many Leo women look great in backless dresses. For a woman who thrives on making dramatic entrances, showing off a little of your backside could help you make your exits just as memorable.

WHO TO WEAR

John Galliano is the undisputed king of runway drama. Despite the theatrics that have overshadowed some of his fashion shows, he continues to be the most brilliantly creative person working in the fashion business today. His designs for both his signature label and the house of Christian Dior are made for women who thrive in the spotlight. But underneath the pomp and splendor of his extravagant catwalk creations lies some of the world's most well-crafted clothing. Galliano is both an artist and an impeccable tailor, and his tremendous craftsmanship is evident in the dramatic complexity of every garment he creates. You, Leo, have the soul of Galliano, and for this reason you should truly delight in the spectacular artistry of the world's most magnificent designer.

JOHN GALLIANO

There are also other labels that suit you well. Thierry Mugler is one of the fashion world's most clever and inventive minds, and many of his designs are theatrical masterpieces. Alexander McQueen designs incredibly creative, dramatic clothing for both his own label and the house of Givenchy. Yves Saint Laurent virtually rewrote the rules of fashion in the last half of the twentieth century, and his signature label's garments can be very complementary to the well-heeled Leo woman. Unfortunately, another thing these designers have in common with Galliano is that much of what they design is prohibitively expensive for the average woman. But don't worry about that, Leo, because you know you're not the average woman. Just watch the runway shows and check out the designers' looks in fashion magazines. Your own creativity should allow you to re-create any look you want. And, as every Leo woman should know, it's not what you wear that makes you look fabulous but rather how you wear it. With your brazen

Leonine attitude, you could wear a burlap sack and still look like a luminary.

WHAT TO AVOID

Some of the best-dressed Leo women are able to wear dramatic clothing every moment of every day. But there are also plenty of badly dressed Leo women who don't have the common sense to know when to tone down the theatrics. They dress in costumes instead of outfits, not realizing that there is a difference between the two. Despite the fact that you are one of the few signs that operates well outside of the traditional fashion establishment, always dressing in costumes can make you look like a buffoon. If you are planning on making people laugh, do it with a brilliant, comedic performance and not by wearing foolishly theatrical outfits when and where they don't belong.

The other type of badly dressed Leo woman never tries to be the superstar she was born to be. She dresses in boring, pedestrian looks that make her appear like just another face in the crowd. Although being born under a fixed sign makes it tough for you to break out of a rut, having the sun as your ruling planet gives you strength and vitality that no other sign possesses. Don't let that power go to waste by adopting a personal style that eclipses your creativity. You were put on this earth to shine, Leo, and you can shine in any outfit you wear. Just decide for yourself if you want to be a blazing supernova or an imperceptible glimmer in a star-filled sky.

HAIR AND MAKEUP

Many Leos are preoccupied with their hair, so it's quite likely that you change your hairstyle more often than other people. But this shouldn't be a problem for you, because the rule of thumb for your hair is to break all the rules. Wear it short or wear it long. Wear it up or wear it down. Color it, streak it, perm it, or cut it all off and start all over again. Just have fun with it, and find yourself a stylist with an open mind and a sense of adventure (a Sagittarius, perhaps). Don't be afraid to put on a wig once in a while, either. Wigs and hair extensions have come a long way in the last few years, and the quality of the products available today is impressive. A great wig can be the crowning achievement to any fabulous outfit the queen of the zodiac chooses to wear. Have some fun, Leo, and please don't get caught donning the same tired hairdo year after year after year.

Being ruled by the sun influences some Leo women to become sun worshipers. There's nothing in the world that can make you feel sexier than a good, dark tan. It's your skin, and you should do what you want, but take this word of advice: Don't go crying to anyone in thirty years because the leathery skin on your face has you looking like an old football. Remember that the sign of Leo rules the circulatory system. So if you want a healthy glow to your complexion, maybe you should get some cardiovascular exercise and forget about tanning.

The sky is the limit as far as your makeup is concerned. You should rejoice in the fact that cosmetics allow you to portray every facet of your Leonine personality. Wearing makeup can make you feel unrestrained by giving you the freedom to create a new visage every time you put yourself together. You can use subtle, muted tones to transform yourself into a waifish ingenue. You can use bright red lipstick and false eyelashes to become a 1950s screen goddess. Or you can use a dramatic mix of high-contrast colors to turn yourself into a man-eating vamp. You can do whatever you want to do. Just remember to put in the effort required to learn how to apply your cosmetics properly, or your crude creative efforts could make you look like a circus clown rather than a cover girl. Purchase fashion magazines on a regular basis, and pay attention to the articles on makeup application. And don't get stuck in a rut by wearing the same old color palette that some know-it-all salesclerk once suggested. Not only is a diverse selection of colors and products in your makeup bag recommended but it is also your astrological birthright. You are the one who calls the shots, Leo, and don't ever forget it.

ACCESSORIES

Although hats have not really been in fashion since the 1960s, that does not mean a woman like you won't look stylish in a hat. Because barely anyone wears hats nowadays, they are probably the single most dramatic accessory you can add to your wardrobe. They are like the icing on the cake for the fabulously decorated Leo woman. Crown yourself with whatever makes you feel majestic. A classic felt fedora looks great with dark sunglasses and a trench coat. A chic beret can bring a tired turtleneck back to life. Feathers can make any outfit into a party outfit. But don't despair if you can't find inexpensive hats in retail stores, because many vintage boutiques are filled with the most exquisite hats. Just take to the time to shop around, Leo, and don't be too proud to buy something beautiful just because it's secondhand. And forget barrettes and headbands. Keep your hair off your face with some strategically placed sunglasses.

A fabulous woman like you also should be carrying a fabulous purse. Don't go picking out the most boring Coach bag in the store just because the salesperson tells you it's a classic. How about something in alligator, ostrich, or leopard print? Maybe even a fur purse. Make a statement about the kind of woman you are by carrying a handbag that doesn't match your shoes. Just be sure you're not hauling around something that doesn't add a little drama to your look. The same advice applies to any other accessories you wear. A Leo woman can never have too many feather boas. Also, gold jewelry and precious stones suit you perfectly, regardless of what is in fashion. And remember, no matter how dull current styles may be, a woman who is dripping with diamonds always looks brilliant.

SOME ADDITIONAL TIPS TO HELP YOU CREATE YOUR OWN COSMIC STYLE

✧ Spicy Oriental fragrances suit a Leo woman's taste for the exotic.

✧ An opulent wedding dress with an open back will suit you perfectly. Carry a bouquet of dramatic gloriosa lilies.

✧ Gold lamé, rich velvet, and other dramatic fabrics will suit your Leo style at the beach. You probably weren't planning on swimming, anyway.

✧ Exotic lingerie will go a long way in your boudoir. Just for fun, get yourself a pair of those high-heeled, maribou-trimmed bedroom slippers, too.

✧ Remember that "Casual Friday" does not mean "Break-All-the-Rules Friday."

✧ Hot nail polish colors will appeal to your fiery sense of style.

✧ Remember to put a little extra thought into choosing shoes. You have the tendency to always look up, and you can overlook the importance of your footwear.

✧ The only accessory you'll want to bring to the gym is a hunky personal trainer.

✧ Cultivate good posture, because you won't look like the queen of the zodiac with a hunched back and sloping shoulders. Your bearing must always be regal.

A FEW WOMEN WHO — FOR BETTER OR WORSE — EXEMPLIFY TRUE LEO STYLE

Jacqueline Kennedy Onassis: July 28

If America ever had a queen of its own, that queen was Jackie O. She virtually reinvented the role of First Lady in the 1960s, and she became the most fashionable woman in the world. With her chic designer outfits, and those big sunglasses perched on her head in typical Leo style, she was the brightest star of her generation.

Martha Stewart: August 3

Martha Stewart may be the world's foremost domestic goddess, but there is nothing divine about the way she dresses. It would be a good thing if she applied some of her innate Leonine craftiness to her incredibly tired appearance.

Lucille Ball: August 6

Early in her career Lucille Ball starred in some movies with her hair dyed blond. But when she colored it flame red her mane became her most distinctive feature, and soon she was the most famous redhead in the world. Like the typical Leo star, Lucille Ball defined herself with a look that everyone would notice.

Whitney Houston: August 9

The pop diva Whitney Houston dresses in gorgeous, theatrical clothes, like the Leo superstar she was born to be. But the one element that defines her Leo look most characteristically is her frequently updated hairstyle. The best-dressed Leo women are never content to look the same from one moment to the next.

Madonna: August 16

When you consider that Madonna is a Leo, it's no surprise that the world's most stylish woman also makes all the worst-dressed lists. The reason is this: We're all jealous because we know that we could never get away with looking so spectacular. She is the most dazzling woman in the world, and everyone should aspire to have just a fraction of her self-assurance.

CHAPTER SIX

VIRGO
THE VIRGIN

August 23–September 22

WHAT MAKES YOU A VIRGO

The worst thing about having high standards is trying to live up to those standards yourself. This is the plight of the Virgo woman. You are the standard-bearer of the zodiac. You possess a keen, analytical mind, and others call on you when they want to bring order to chaos. You are the ultimate employee, not only inclined to render excellent service but also capable of creating a work environment where others thrive. Your critical acumen is legendary, and people request your opinion regularly because they know that even if your conclusions are contrary to theirs, you are logical and well-informed. However, Virgo, this innate talent for qualifying and quantifying everything around you is rarely applied where it would matter the most: on yourself. You are the greatest critic in the world, but you often let yourself down.

The reason you expect so much from everyone else is that your ruling planet is Mercury. Mercury also rules over Gemini, giving members of that sign a talent for external communication. But you feel the influence of the planet internally: It's all in your head, Virgo. Many of you are remarkably intelligent, and even if you are not intellectual, you likely have a more cerebral orientation than most people. Your brain works systematically, organizing details the way a librarian organizes books. Everything inside your head is categorized correctly and on the right shelf, and you never have a difficult time locating something you're searching for. Unfortunately, Mercury's influence also causes you to get so caught up in the minute details of everyday life that you neglect significant matters even when they scream for your attention. Occasionally you lose touch with the big picture altogether, and then you end up in a situation that you are far too bright to be involved in. Mercury may have given you brains, Virgo, but many of you suffer from a complete lack of common sense.

Along with Taurus and Capricorn, Virgo is one of the earth signs. The no-nonsense, practical nature of the earth element counteracts a few of the more undesirable Mercurial aspects of your personality, such as immaturity. In addition, Virgo is a mutable sign, allowing you to adapt well to changing circumstances. Together with the influence of Mercury, these factors give rise to typical Virgo character traits. Expressed in a positive manner, these traits include modesty, adaptability, diligence, serviceability, and an outstanding organizational ability. Expressed in a negative manner, Virgo qualities include shyness, anxiousness, peevishness, a tendency toward self-delusion, and an excessively critical nature. At your most negative, you tend to disguise low-self-esteem issues behind a critical facade, so it is imperative that you learn to express yourself positively. Even though you're good at articulating the shortcomings of others, you shouldn't make criticism your full-time job. You are the zodiac's true perfectionist, but finding fault in everything is truly obnoxious. When you take the time to evaluate yourself—the way you act, the way you dress, the way you look—you'll discover that the effort you've put into critiquing others may have been more judiciously spent on yourself.

YOUR KEYWORD

The keyword that best defines the well-dressed Virgo woman is *exquisite*. Despite your intellectual propensity, you are a rather down-to-earth person. In a way you are much like the clay that artists sculpt with. There is nothing remarkable about clay in its raw state; it is heavy, shapeless, and crude. But in your hands clay can become something quite exquisite. It can be fit into a mold, where it takes on the character of its environment. It can be sculpted into a freestanding masterpiece that inspires awe with its beauty. It can be anything you want it to be, if you are willing to put in the time and effort it takes to master the medium. Think of yourself as both the medium and the artisan when it comes to fashion. You can mold and shape yourself into whatever you want to be, but you will not create a masterpiece until you have made an effort to study the art form. Being fashionable is an art form, and looking exquisite takes both talent and effort. If you apply yourself studiously, Virgo, there is no doubt that you will be able to master the art of style.

YOUR THREE RULES TO DRESS BY

1: Evaluate

The fact that Virgos are critically inclined gets repeated so often it begins to sound like a cliché. But, as any Virgo would tell you, there's nothing wrong with a cliché. Virgos love to categorize and evaluate everything around them. With nothing more than a passing glance, they will assess anything they can, eagerly offering their analysis. However, this tendency toward superficiality must be checked. In your desire to label everything, you often forget to turn your critical eye on yourself. You need to take a long, hard look at your own sense of style, then seriously evaluate the contents of your closet. Unless every detail meets your high standards, don't consider yourself among the best-dressed. No one is impressed by a critic with no credentials, so hold your tongue until you look like the fashion expert you claim to be. The only person you need to impress is yourself, so spend the time to evaluate what it will take to do that.

2: Plan

Once you've succeeded in evaluating your own style, you can begin to do whatever is necessary to join the ranks of the well-dressed. Virgos are the master planners of the zodiac, so developing a plan to improve your wardrobe should be second nature to you. Whether it takes a visit to a stylist who can assist you in defining your characteristic look or simply a shopping trip for the items that will complete your wardrobe, you must plan to do it. Moreover, you must plan to make wardrobe building a habit. Shopping in impulsive binges or only shopping when the mood strikes you will get you into trouble. You are at your methodical best when you are forced into a routine—this same quality is what makes you such a valuable employee. So plan to shop. First, pick a certain day of the week for your regular shopping excursion. Next, decide exactly what your wardrobe needs. Finally, go out and get it. When you stick to a plan, Virgo, you can make looking good part of your routine.

3: Reflect

Many Virgos are remarkably self-deluded. The most striking example of Virgo self-delusion is seen in the character of Blanche DuBois in Tennessee Williams's classic play *A*

Streetcar Named Desire. Blanche is a Virgo—she says so her-self. She's also sort of crazy and completely unaware of how truly pathetic she is. Like many other Virgos, she has no apti-tude for self-reflection. When she looks into a mirror she does not see the tragic heroine everyone else sees. Every Virgo woman needs to develop a capacity for self-reflection. If you look into the mirror and can't see the same person others see, then you have a problem. You must learn to be completely hon-est with yourself so that you can view your reflection objectively. Subjectivity is in your nature: That's what makes you such a first-rate critic. But self-delusion is also in your nature. Once you admit it is, the image you see in the mirror will become a much clearer reflection of who you really are.

SPECIFICS: WHAT TO WEAR

✦ Being an earth sign makes Virgos fond of earthy colors. The shades that suit you best are in the middle of the earth-tone spectrum. Medium browns, taupes, and earthy greens look exquisite on the well-dressed Virgo woman.

✦ White also looks stunning on you. You can get away with wearing black, too. In general, a closet full of simple neu-tral tones can help you avoid making mistakes when you are coordinating wardrobe pieces. Let simplicity be your maxim when choosing colors to wear, and don't allow yourself to get caught up in trends by wearing the so-called "in" color.

✧ While many women rely on a closet full of wardrobe pieces they can mix and match to create several outfits, you are not the zodiac's greatest separates dresser. In fact, you can do yourself a favor by buying the whole look. Many of the best apparel manufacturers design outfits—suits, dresses, and so on—that have been created to stand alone rather than coordinated with other garments. These outfits are beautiful, and the only accessory they require is a beautiful woman like you to wear them. This foolproof style of dressing suits you perfectly.

✧ Many truly fashionable people consider dressing in classic apparel taking the easy way out. But it doesn't have to be. A Virgo woman's flair for fashion lies in her ability to look impeccable when those around her look like fashion victims. Don't equate an aversion to trends with a lack of personal style. You've got fashion sense to spare, Virgo, even if your own personal style whispers rather than screams.

✧ Looking exquisite does require maintenance. Your clothing ought to be clean, pressed, and free from undue wear or other imperfections. You are the perfectionist of the zodiac, and your apparel must reflect that fact.

✧ Virgo women normally express no preference between pants and skirts. However, most well-heeled Virgo women acknowledge that suits are the cornerstones of their wardrobes. Many also profess a fondness for dresses. Coat dresses, which combine the look of a suit with the simplicity of a dress, are ideal Virgo outfits.

✧ People born under an earth sign generally have a rather material nature. For this reason many Virgo women can become label whores, and they wear designer clothing because they believe that status can be bought. Get real, Virgo! Some of the most stylish people in the world buy their clothing in secondhand stores and consignment boutiques. Always remember that there is a difference between buying a look and looking good.

✧ Natural fabrics suit you well. Cotton, silk, linen, and wool all are good choices for you.

✧ Many women shun wool because they once owned a poor-quality wool sweater that made them itchy. The key to wearing wool is products that are soft, well-crafted, suited to your climate, and lined where they are supposed to be lined. Even in the middle of summer, a lined tropical wool suit can be a perfect addition to your wardrobe.

✧ Simple fabrics suit you better than complicated materials. Avoid a lot of lace, eyelet, beadwork, and sequins. Shaggy knitwear or garments with dangling pieces of fabric are bad choices for you as well. Any extraneous material on your clothing should be simple. Virgos are great with details, but don't ever believe that intricately detailed clothing will suit you better than simplicity.

✧ Leather and suede garments can be attractive to your earthy sense of style. They also can make you feel especially sexy. Leather pants come in and out of fashion frequently, so consider getting yourself a pair next time they're in.

✧ While you should avoid most patterns, there are a few designs that suit you well. Small-scale geometric patterns can add a little flair to your otherwise subdued look. Houndstooth or Prince of Wales plaid will appeal to your love of detail, but avoid garish tartans and other complicated patterns. Botanical prints may appeal to you, too, but only in their simplest form. A small-scale floral print on a lovely summer dress will make you feel lovely yourself.

✧ Having fickle Mercury as your ruling planet can make you envious of those who dress in a far more fashion-forward style than you. However, dressing in trendy styles is not your style, Virgo. Always put common sense ahead of your desire to splurge on impractical trendy items. If you can convince yourself to think twice before making a purchase, your urge to keep up with the trends will usually pass before you've made a big mistake.

WHO TO WEAR

The designer who exemplifies all the best—and the worst—of true Virgo style is Miuccia Prada. She is one of the fashion world's foremost intellectuals. Both her Prada and Miu

Miu lines are designed in a manner that seems calculated and cerebral. Yet there is an uncomplicated beauty to many of her collections that appeals to a Virgo woman's love of simplicity. But she also makes all the typical mistakes that a poorly dressed Virgo woman makes. Prada's obsessive flair for detail sometimes makes her clothing appear unwearable. Instead of simply accepting the aesthetic purity of her initial design, she compromises her creations with foolish, trend-oriented details: Her mirror-tiled dresses are just one example. There is no doubt that she is one of the most talented designers in the world, but she must learn to accept that there is no shame in being uncomplicated.

Miuccia Prada

Another line that should appeal to you is Club Monaco. Originally created by the Canadian designer Alfred Sung, the Club Monaco label has generated a lot of buzz in the fashion world for its consistently simple yet fashionable attire. Many critics claim that the label relies on inexpensive knockoffs of designer looks to remain successful, but anyone who has shopped at Club Monaco for years knows that this is not the case. Club Monaco is a gift from the heavens for anyone who can't afford designer prices. There are many other labels that suit you well by providing those stand-alone outfits that make your wardrobe complete. Max Mara, for instance, creates gorgeous apparel that can make you look both simple and fashionable. And without the high-end designer price tag, it appeals to the practical side of your nature.

WHAT TO AVOID

Badly dressed Virgo women generally fall into two categories. The first is the Virgo woman who wears nothing but designer labels. There is nothing wrong with wanting to wear beautiful designer clothing. However, there is something wrong with wearing labels simply because you believe that a label earns you some sort of social status. Just look around you, Virgo. There are as many hideously dressed rich women out there carrying Louis Vuitton purses as there are poor women who look like a million bucks. Possessing straight-off-the-rack style is like having no style at all. Learn to wear what looks good on you, and always wear the kind of clothing that lets other people know what you're about. If you don't want to look like a fashion victim, don't rely on designer labels to define your character.

The other type of badly dressed Virgo woman is the detail-obsessed woman. Sometimes a Virgo woman can lose touch with the big picture because she allows minute details to command her attention. When this tendency affects the way she dresses, the result is a woman who goes overboard with detail. Every square inch of fabric she wears is covered with sequins, beads, patterns, appliqués, or embroidery. There are fabulous designers who have made careers by producing richly detailed clothing: Emanuel Ungaro and Valentino are masters of fine detail. But most of their ornate clothing is better suited to a red-carpet reception than to everyday life. Unless you're planning to attend an awards show every night of the week, try to go easy on the details, Virgo. Simplicity becomes you. It's in the stars.

HAIR AND MAKEUP

A fresh-faced, uncomplicated look suits you best, Virgo. But styles change, and sometimes heavier makeup is de rigueur. Just try to strike a balance between your love of simplicity and the current trends. For inspiration look to the classical beauty of the actress Ingrid Bergman. Unlike many of her screen goddess contemporaries, Bergman was able to star in several films while wearing what appears to be a fraction of the makeup they wore. She was beauty personified in a simple yet exquisite manner. That is your look, Virgo: simple, exquisite.

Another matter you need to consider when purchasing cosmetics is your tendency to splurge on labels. Designer cosmetic lines can be both fashionable and wonderful to wear. But they also can be overpriced. Since you've got a good head on your shoulders, take the time to investigate the products you purchase. If you can get away with inexpensive products that perform just as well as the higher-profile lines, you should be wearing them. Sometimes a lipstick is just a lipstick.

Like your makeup, your hairstyle should be rather uncomplicated. A good cut that allows for some versatility while styling is something that you must invest in. A good hairstylist is going to cost you, Virgo, but you should never attempt to put a price on a well-informed opinion. The reason for this is your tendency toward self-delusion. You could think that you look great when everyone else is thinking, Doesn't she own a mirror? You must commit to paying for a hairstylist you can trust. Look for someone who is blunt and won't candy-coat the truth. Find a salon where no one walks out until she looks fabulous. If it costs you more, just deal with it. You wear your hair every day, so be sure you have a style that you'll want to wear every day. Your entire look depends upon it.

ACCESSORIES

Even though many of you are obsessively orderly, there are just as many of you who only aspire to be organized. For instance, Virgos have the messiest purses in the zodiac. You try too hard to be well-prepared and consequently carry far too much. The result is an overstuffed satchel with about as much aesthetic appeal as a homeless woman's shopping cart. You must clean out your purse, Virgo! First, get rid of most of the garbage in it, then find yourself a bag you can't fit that much into. All you really need is a little money, a lipstick, some ID, and maybe a tampon. Once you've downsized your bag, purchase yourself a good daily journal. Writing down your appointments and obsessively planning your life for the next several weeks will help to distract you from the symptoms of large-purse withdrawal.

The type of purse that suits you best is small, simple, and

well-designed. The Prada nylon bag that helped launch that company's success is a good choice for you. A classic Louis Vuitton monogram bag will appeal to you, too. You like rather simple shoes as well. Even though brown leather shoes may be especially appealing to your earthy sense of style, make sure that you have just as many black shoes in your closet. You likely have a fondness for masculine loafers that can be worn with suits. This style of footwear suits you well, but don't ever forget that a sexy pair of high heels can take you places loafers will never go. Your hosiery is generally well-selected and appropriate for the garments you pair it with. Your jewelry is usually exquisite, and you rarely wear anything cheap or garish. In addition, a well-dressed Virgo woman generally avoids garish hair hardware. As with other accessories, you seem to have a less-is-more approach when it comes adorning your hairstyle. Keep it that way, Virgo. Don't let yourself get hung up on the petty details, or before you know it you'll be decked out like a Christmas tree.

SOME ADDITIONAL TIPS TO HELP YOU CREATE YOUR OWN COSMIC STYLE

✧ Virgo rules over the stomach. If you have a flat stomach— and a little more confidence than the other Virgo girls— show it off in a midriff-baring top.

✧ A classically cut, athletic swimsuit will appeal to you.

✧ Sensual, earthy, green perfumes suit you well. Fragrances that smell good enough to eat are especially attractive on you.

✧ If you are getting married, try to avoid an excessively detailed dress that is difficult to wear. Too much beading or lacework can make you feel quite uncomfortable. Carry a mixed bouquet of small flowers when you walk down the aisle.

✧ No one wears white better than the Virgo woman. For this reason, sexy white undergarments and lingerie look great on you.

✧ The earthy side of your personality could have you sleeping in soft flannel or exquisite silk. But, more likely, you enjoy sleeping in the buff. You like to wear nothing when you're all alone.

✧ Eastern cultures may influence the way you dress. The simplicity of the Japanese aesthetic is especially alluring to you.

✧ Long fingernails do not suit you. Keep them on the short side, and paint them a subdued color. The French manicure is a classic Virgo look.

✧ If your co-workers think you're a little uptight, use "Casual Friday" to show them just how easygoing you can be.

✧ Virgos are prone to health problems caused by compulsive behavior. Many of these bad habits can profoundly affect your physical appearance. Try to get professional help if that's what it takes to adopt a healthier lifestyle.

✧ You could be wearing years of anxiety on your face, Virgo, so a face-lift could make you very happy. However, not worrying so much could make you just as happy—and it may also help relax those creases on your brow.

A FEW WOMEN WHO— FOR BETTER OR WORSE— EXEMPLIFY TRUE VIRGO STYLE

Claudia Schiffer: August 25

The Teutonic supermodel Claudia Schiffer looks great in everything she wears—she's just that beautiful. But she looks extraordinarily beautiful when she wears white. Like a typical Virgo woman, she is at her most heavenly when she dons this quintessential Virgo color.

Shania Twain: August 28

Although her down-home charm has made her a millionaire, the singer Shania Twain's personal style is still more trailer park than Park Avenue. She is undeniably gorgeous, but she looks anything but gorgeous in her tacky evening wear and yokel duds. Evidently, she is missing the most important accessory a Virgo woman can own: a full-length mirror.

Ingrid Bergman: August 29

How could Ingrid Bergman ever look bad? In an era when every actress was dressed to the nines, Bergman's natural beauty managed to shine through the layers of makeup and clothing. In true Virgo style, she was simply exquisite in an unpretentious and uncomplicated way.

Cameron Diaz: August 30

The actress Cameron Diaz looks her best when she goes easy on the makeup. As the girl next door in *There's Something About Mary* (1998), she was so sweet and lovable that she attracted three stalkers simultaneously. While that isn't a goal most women should aspire to, Virgos should aspire to be just as lovely as Cameron Diaz by easing up on the cosmetics.

Sophia Loren: September 20

Sophia Loren is truly incomparable. The secret to her perfection lies in her aversion to trends, the simplicity of her wardrobe, and her reliance upon suits. She can turn every head in the room by wearing nothing more than a simple skirt, a matching jacket, and a pair of shoes. By simplifying your own look, you can plan to look great, too.

LIBRA
THE SCALES

September 23–October 22

WHAT MAKES YOU A LIBRA

Looking good should come easy to you, Libra. It is a well-known fact that you have the best taste in the zodiac. You have a refined aesthetic sense and a strong desire to be in elegant surroundings. You thrive in a tasteful, harmonious environment, and you feel tranquil and content when you are in the presence of beauty. However, your taste for the finer things in life is somewhat extrinsic: You truly appreciate the beauty that surrounds you, yet you often neglect to consider the role you play in your environment. You have the tendency to distance yourself from the world around you, becoming an observer of events rather than an active participant. The reason for this is your passivity. You are remarkably passive—many have accused you of being lazy—and you usually prefer to blend into the background. It's not shyness, or even modesty for that matter, that makes you act this way. You're just too laid-back. You might be the most tasteful girl in the zodiac, Libra, but what good is good taste when you're too laid-back to exercise it?

Venus, the planet of love, beauty, and harmony, rules over your sign. You can thank Venus for endowing you with your highly developed aesthetic sense. But you can also blame her for your passivity. Venus hates a fight. In mythology she was the goddess of love, and her purpose was to bring people together. For this reason the sign of Libra is associated with relationships. You crave companionship, and harmonious personal relationships mean as much to you as a harmonious, beautiful environment. But attracting the sorts of relationships you desire can be difficult because of your passive nature. Venus has endowed you with the ability to be breathtakingly beautiful, but many of you just don't put in the effort that looking attractive requires. You have the loveliest planet in the zodiac on your side, but she's also the laziest planet. Her influence is both a blessing and a curse.

While the influence of Venus has a profound effect on you, it does not act alone in defining the characteristics of your sign. Libra is a cardinal sign. The cardinal quality grants you the ability to be straightforward. Libra is also one of the air signs, like Gemini and Aquarius. Being born under the air element gives you an intellectual bent and the ability to distinguish between rational thought and emotional impulse. When the influence of Venus is blended with the cardinal quality and the air element, typical Libra character traits emerge. Positive Libran characteristics can include elegance, refinement, perceptiveness, kindness, and a natural skill for diplomacy. Negative traits can include laziness, indecisiveness, timidity, a codependent nature, and an inability to confront your problems. You must learn to assert yourself and show off those positive traits more often. Even though your aesthetic sense is outstanding, no one will know it unless you put in the effort that it takes to look your best. Overcoming your passivity is your biggest challenge, a challenge that you must accept. You are born with the potential to be extraordinarily attractive, but potential alone does not make a beautiful woman.

YOUR KEYWORD

Picture the air that defines your sign as the peaceful air within the eye of a hurricane. A hurricane is a violent clash of air under low pressure with air under high pressure. But in the center of the hurricane is the eye: a spot where the pressure is perfectly balanced. The result is a placid oasis that seems to defy the nature of its chaotic environment. You are like the eye of a hurricane because you are able to maintain balance and remain composed in intense situations. Accordingly, *balance* is the keyword you must remember every time you get dressed. As the scales that represent your sign imply, you require balance in your life. You desire harmony in your environment in much the same way you crave balance in your mental state. Not only are you a born peacemaker but Venus also gives you a tranquil, kindhearted nature that inspires the same qualities in others. Like the goddess Venus, Librans can elicit peace and harmony in their environment by virtue of their serene appearance.

YOUR THREE RULES TO DRESS BY

1: Be Patient

If there was only one reason to be thankful about your passive nature, that reason would be your uncanny ability to sit back and examine a situation patiently. Many of you have been accused of being spineless or incapable of making a decision. While that may be true of some of you, many of you are great at decision making—just incredibly slow to arrive at a conclusion. You think everything through thoroughly, and you rarely commit to a situation unless you've examined it yourself. Although an inability to act on impulses may make you feel that you are too cautious, it's nothing to be ashamed of. In fact, it makes you a better shopper than most people. Instead of traipsing through a mall and buying whatever you grab, you patiently think your purchases through. A well-dressed Libra woman sits down at the start of a new season and decides exactly what she needs to make her wardrobe complete. Then she patiently peruses the stores in order to get what she wants. By being composed she always looks great, because her patience prevents her from make regrettable mistakes.

2: Refine

Beauty is in the eye of the beholder. But certain looks do have a more universal appeal than others. Many women wear clothing that isn't particularly chic, yet it has a refined quality that makes them appear elegant and sophisticated. Their wardrobes consist of well-made garments in luxurious materials that withstand the test of time. The well-dressed Libra woman has mastered this "refined" look. Rather than spending her money on trend-oriented pieces, she sticks to more traditional looks. She has a closet full of outfits that defy the current styles, yet there is nothing unfashionable about her appearance. She can keep an outfit for years, then wear it as if it were new. There is a timeless elegance to the well-dressed Libra woman that is aesthetically appealing regardless of the prevailing trends. By refining her look, she defines herself as someone who knows that being stylish doesn't require buying a sense of style.

3: Attract

Being ruled by Venus gives Libra women a romantic nature. However, you're not a dreamy romantic, like a Pisces girl. Instead, you are a practical romantic, and you understand that attracting an admirer requires more than just fantasizing about love. The most attractive Libra women work hard to learn how to utilize the tools of the beauty trade—clothes, cosmetics, fragrances, accessories—to present themselves in a manner that others find irresistible. Looking attractive is an essential element of Libra style, because attracting harmonious relationships is essential to your well-being. Too many badly dressed Libra women undervalue the power of physical attraction. There is no shame in admitting that looking good is important to you. If you use your looks to draw people into your world, you're one step closer to showing them how beautiful you are on the inside, too.

SPECIFICS: WHAT TO WEAR

- ✧ Airy colors suit you well. Light colors, such as pastel shades, are especially becoming on a Libra woman. It is likely that you have a fondness for the softest blues and greens.

- ✧ Colors with a hint of metallic luster will also look great on you. The soft shine of champagne colors or pearly gray shades appeal to you.

- ✧ Intense colors should be avoided unless you wear them in a monochromatic or tone-on-tone scheme. The balanced look that defines a well-dressed Libra woman cannot be achieved by wearing blocks of color or high-contrast color combinations.

- ✧ Your primary concern when you are getting dressed should be to elongate your silhouette. The simplest way to accomplish this is to wear a single color from head to toe.

✧ The lean, elegant geometry that defined the Art Deco movement in the twenties and thirties is a classic Libra look. Not only was the style of clothing from this period modern and sophisticated but it also was very complementary to a woman's body. It emphasized height, giving the wearer a more statuesque appearance. It was sexy and feminine without being terribly revealing. No retro style suits you better.

✧ Lean pantsuits will appeal to you. Longer jackets worn over straight-legged pants can add length to your look, but very short jackets should be avoided.

✧ Slim skirts look better on you than A-line styles or anything voluminous. Short skirts are okay, but they must be worn with the appropriate hosiery to lengthen your shape.

✧ Loose-fitting garments do not suit you. Regardless of your size or body type, you ought to wear clothing that fits closely. There are many tricks you can use to disguise your figure flaws, but wearing ill-fitting clothing is not among them.

✧ Many Libra women live in pants. Suit yourself, if wearing pants makes you happy. Just remember that a long, lean dress can make you look slim and feel beautiful.

✧ The one garment every Libra woman should put to use in her wardrobe is the bodysuit. In the 1980s the designer Donna Karan made a name for herself by reintroducing the bodysuit as an essential wardrobe piece. Worn under a suit, it adds length to a woman's figure while emphasizing her curves. No piece of clothing complements a Libra woman more than a beautiful bodysuit. If the current styles allow you to wear one, you should be wearing one.

✧ Finely woven, well-crafted fabrics look better on you than anything bulky. Wear the smoothest silks, the finest cashmere, or the most intricate lace. Any fabric that is luxurious appeals to your decadent nature.

✧ Like other luxury fabrics, leather, suede, camel hair, fur, and exotic animal hides may appeal to you. If you don't mind wearing fur, a full-length, champagne-colored mink coat will make you feel like a million bucks.

✧ If you can't afford a mink coat or you choose not to wear fur, buy yourself a classic beige trench coat. Choose a style that is lean, and avoid large shoulder pads. A beautiful trench coat is a quintessential Libra garment.

✧ You must exercise caution when choosing patterned clothing. Vertical pinstripes look great on you. But the well-dressed Libra woman never wears horizontal stripes, regardless of how thin she is. Geometric patterns may appeal to you, too, but only in their simplest form.

✧ If avoiding patterned clothing altogether seems boring to you, try to add some interest to your wardrobe with beaded garments. Intricate beadwork patterns can be refined and elegant without being tacky. When you want to dress up, an exquisitely beaded outfit can make you look gorgeous.

✧ Being an air sign allows you to get away with some interesting fabric choices. Sheer or see-through fabrics will add some sex appeal to your wardrobe. They also can support spectacular beadwork. Loose knits, as long as they are not too chunky, also appeal to your airy nature.

✧ Although Libra is considered a masculine sign, Venus endows you with the power to use your feminine wiles to your advantage. In a corporate environment, your straightforward manner and professional looks can take you places that have traditionally been dominated by men. The Libra look is very office-friendly. But outside the office your good taste can make you look attractive and feminine without looking sleazy. So don't waste your time complaining about double standards, Libra. Learn to view your astrological gender as something that allows you to experience the best of both worlds.

WHO TO WEAR

The designs of Donna Karan epitomize the Libra look. Like most successful American designers, she has built her fashion empire on sportswear. But what sets her apart from the competition is her love of modern elegance. She creates clothing that is simple without being plain. Whether she accomplishes this by using rich fabrics or by adding luxurious details, she manages to produce a signature line that is opulent without being ostentatious. She also emphasizes length. There is a lean, architectural quality to her best creations that can make a woman appear statuesque regardless of her physical stature. Karan seems to have a gift for adding height to a woman's figure without adding mass. You appreciate this—as an air sign you don't like to be weighed down by your clothes. Unlike many of her male counterparts, Karan also knows what makes a woman feel attractive because she wears the clothes she designs. You, Libra, are at your best when you look lean, elegant, and attractive. That is why the designs of Donna Karan are made just for you.

Donna Karan

Several other designers make clothing that appeals to your sophisticated sense of style. In the seventies, Halston made a career out of designing long, lean looks. Randolph Duke designs stunning evening wear in the tradition of Halston. The same can be said for the gorgeous dresses by the Badgley Mischka label. But if less formal clothing is what you're after, you should have no problem finding outfits that suit you. The French line Celine balances the ease of American sportswear with typical Parisian opulence. Since Michael Kors took over the design duties at Celine, he has revolutionized the label, making sophisticated luxury both beautiful and easygoing—just like the well-dressed Libra woman. All these designer lines can be a bit pricey, but it is a price that you ought to be willing to pay. As mentioned before, you can wear outfits for years, regardless of the current craze. You have a bearing that is natural and elegant, and you can defy trends by simply being beautiful. So spend your money on clothes you'll want to wear for years. Let "quality over quantity" be your maxim. You were born to wear beautiful clothes, Libra. It's in the stars.

WHAT TO AVOID

The worst-dressed Libra women are too easygoing for their own good. They don't appreciate all that fashion has to offer them, and they don't live up to the potential of their sign. Many people complain that the fashion industry sets standards of beauty that are impossible to live up to. But that simply isn't true. Fashion evens the playing field by giving us all the chance to present ourselves in the best possible light. It allows us to disguise our perceived figure flaws. It allows us to change the look we were born with by providing tools that can make our appearance more to our own liking. There is nothing shallow about wanting to look better, because looking good on the outside can make us feel glorious on the inside. Every Libra woman ought to recognize that making an effort to look good is important. You have an unparalleled aesthetic sense, but that in itself does not make you attractive. Strive to become more beautiful and learn to exercise your good taste.

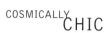
A more specific type of poorly dressed Libra woman is the tacky Libra woman. As mentioned before, many Libra women spend a lot of money on clothing that they can wear for years. Quality is a luxury that you should pay for. But the tacky Libra woman doesn't understand this. She attempts to make herself beautiful by wearing clothing that she considers pretty, even when it is ridiculously gaudy or out-of-date. She wears cheap fabrics that don't stand the test of time. She adorns herself with cheesy accessories that make her look garish rather than stylish. She wears her hair in a style that most people gave up on a decade before, and her makeup palette has been the same for years. If any of this sounds familiar to you, you must learn to exercise your taste more discriminatingly. Your aesthetic sense is not infallible. If you think it is, perhaps you have stepped over the line where tasteful ends and tacky begins.

HAIR AND MAKEUP

More than any other sign in the zodiac, you were born to wear your hair long. Long, straight hair enhances the lean, elegant look that defines you so well. Symmetrical styles, such as center parts, suit you better than asymmetry. But asymmetrical styles can help you to downplay an uneven feature—a crooked nose, for instance. You enjoy looking balanced, even if it takes a little imbalance in your look to achieve that aim. If long hair doesn't suit you, or if you are simply too laid-back to maintain a longer style, try to keep your hair styled in a downward direction as long as it still looks good on you. Big, puffy hair can look comic on you: Your fellow Libran Fran Drescher can attest to that. Very short hair should be avoided, although many older women do look better with their hair shorter and off their faces. Regardless of how you wear your hair, please take care of it. If your roots should have been touched up months ago and your split ends are creeping toward your scalp, then get to a salon. Beauty takes maintenance, Libra. Don't ever forget it.

Makeup is something that you need to invest in. As an air sign, you don't look good in heavy makeup, but you should be wearing something. Foundation is the most important product in your cosmetic bag. A balanced, uniform complexion is important to you. Even if you don't have a great complexion, foundation will help you. Improving your skin-care regime will also allow you to look better. Your easygoing nature may make you the kind of woman who does not put in the time or effort that proper skin care requires. Nothing is going to make you look better than a gorgeous, glowing complexion—so get to work, Libra. As for the rest of your makeup, light colors will appeal to you, as will a little metallic sheen. Airy blues and greens often look good on your eyes, and a little silvery white may suit you, too. Try to avoid bright lip color except for the most traditional reds. Bright fuchsia or brilliant orange are bad choices for you, and too much pink will make you look tacky. You're at your best when you look classy and elegant, so don't leave your house looking like a tart. Cheap is a look that you'll never pull off.

Your ruling planet, Venus, makes you a little more high-maintenance then most other women. The kind of beauty regimen that makes you look beautiful takes a great deal of effort. Take comfort in the fact that when you do put in the effort, you look better than almost anyone else.

ACCESSORIES

You have a taste for the finer things in life, and it's likely that you also have a taste for the finest luxury goods. Never wear cheap jewelry. And even if you can't afford something like a Louis Vuitton handbag, go to a store that sells them and ask a clerk to show you one. Once it's in your hands you'll know exactly why you should have a bag like that. Those shivers up and down your spine don't lie. Regardless of the brand of purse you choose to carry, you probably prefer a long shoulder strap to a shorter handle. Because Libra rules the hips, you should try to carry a small, neutral-colored bag that doesn't draw attention to that area. Unless you're very thin, you can be especially sensitive about your hip region.

An accessory you should learn to love is the high-heeled shoe. Because your signature look depends on lengthening your silhouette, high heels can help you achieve a little more stature. Even if that heel is an inch tall, it's better than no heel at all. Because your sign rules the pelvis, walking in heels normally comes easy to you. Most of you walk in an upright stance with your pelvis tucked slightly inward: the perfect position for standing up straight in your heels. If you can't walk in heels, perhaps you need to evaluate your posture. It's never too late to strengthen your muscles and stand up straight. So make a point of getting some exercise, Libra. Your whole bearing will be improved, and maybe then you'll be able to strut around in those sexy Manolo Blahniks.

SOME ADDITIONAL TIPS TO HELP YOU CREATE YOUR OWN COSMIC STYLE

✧ On your wedding day, a simple satin column will make you look gorgeous. Carry a bouquet of dark red roses down the aisle. Roses are your flower, Libra.

✧ The type of perfume that suits you well is a light floral, applied just as lightly.

✧ Wear something fun on "Casual Friday." You have a social nature, and you enjoy going out with co-workers on Friday evening. A little black dress can take you from daytime to evening without a lot of effort.

✧ A day trip to a salon is recommended whenever you're down in the dumps. Getting pampered will always put you in a good mood.

✧ Because you can be too easygoing, your fingernails may suffer from a lack of maintenance. If this is the case, make regular appointments with a manicurist.

✧ Comfort is very important to you, and you likely enjoy a comfortable bed. In fact, what you wear to bed is less important to you than the bedding itself. Whether you prefer soft cotton flannel sheets or the richest linen bedclothes, you love luxurious bedding.

✧ When you do wear sexy lingerie, you only wear the best. No cheap polyester teddies for you, Libra.

✧ Because you are acutely sensitive about your hip region, you may never wear a swimsuit in public. You ought to spend less time worrying about the size of your hips and more time in the gym. You'll be happy with the results.

A FEW WOMEN WHO— FOR BETTER OR WORSE— EXEMPLIFY TRUE LIBRA STYLE

Heather Locklear: September 25

The lovely Heather Locklear is best known for the trampy-looking characters she has played on TV. How can anyone forget her trashy blond hair and dark roots on *Melrose Place*? But her finest work so far has been her duty as spokesperson for a major beauty products company. With her high-maintenance look, she is Libra charm and elegance personified.

Barbara Walters: September 25

Barbara Walters is not that tall. But in typical Libra fashion, she virtually towers over most women her size. Like any well-dressed Libra woman, she enhances her stature by wearing chic, flattering outfits in monochromatic color schemes.

Janeane Garafolo: September 28

The comic actress Janeane Garafolo has a beautiful face that the camera loves. But off camera she appears too laid-back, and she hardly ever dresses up. In her sloppy, casual clothes she rarely lives up to the potential of her natural beauty.

Gwyneth Paltrow: September 28

No actress has had such a great run in the press as Gwyneth Paltrow. Has anyone ever taken a bad picture of her? Probably not, because in typical Libra style she is always "put together." In tasteful garments that flatter her lean, attractive body, she is on her way to becoming one of Hollywood's most memorable fashion icons.

Sigourney Weaver: October 8

The actress Sigourney Weaver looks her best in the slim, elegant dresses that suit Libra women so well. However, she sometimes gets carried away with trends, and then the press has a field day criticizing her as a fashion victim. All Libra women must learn that the type of clothing you carry off the best is sophisticated, elegant, and never trendy.

SCORPIO
THE SCORPION

October 23–November 21

WHAT MAKES YOU A SCORPIO

Scorpio, you've got a bad reputation. Whether you've earned that reputation is another matter. Your astrological sign is associated with sex, and when people find out that you're a Scorpio, they jump to the conclusion that you are preoccupied with sex. You probably do think about sex a lot, but so does everyone else. However, it's human nature to put other people into categories, and somehow you've been put into a category that makes you feel like you are the most misunderstood girl in the zodiac. Not only are you labeled a sex maniac but your sign is associated with other provocative subjects, including death and the occult. You also have a rather unique ability to conceal your emotions under an icy veneer. Like the typical icy blonde in an Alfred Hitchcock movie, you ought to cultivate this characteristic. An ice princess demeanor appears strangely attractive on you. Scorpio is also represented by a deadly, venomous arachnid. These connections to unpleasant matters have provided you with a reputation that you simply do not deserve. It's tough to be a Scorpio. By having been born under a sign that is feared and maligned, you are guilty by association. But it doesn't have to be that way, Scorpio. Just like everyone else, you have a good side.

Pluto is your ruling planet. In mythology Pluto was the god of the underworld. Having Pluto rule over your sign puts you in touch with the darker side of human nature. You realize that the world you live in isn't all sweetness and light. By recognizing this, you are much more realistic than other people. Unfortunately, others don't view you as realistic: They view you as morose, depressed, or pessimistic. But that simply isn't true. You can be the life of the party if you want to be. You just don't want to be the life of the party if earning that reputation means you have to live with your head up in the clouds. Pluto has opened your eyes to the natural, physical world, and that includes death, birth, sex, violence, and many other subjects people like to sweep under the rug. You know that without darkness there would be no light. Instead of ignoring these things, you accept them as part of your life.

Pluto allows you to comprehend the realities that define your existence.

While having Pluto as your ruling planet may seem like a cross to bear, you can be thankful that it is not the only factor that characterizes your sign. Scorpio is also a water sign, along with Cancer and Pisces. The water element makes you very sensitive. You can trust your emotional responses to situations. In addition, Scorpio is one of the fixed signs. The fixed quality bestows you with a steady, stable nature that makes you seem rather predictable to those who really know you, despite your mysterious demeanor. When the sensate water element is combined with the steadfast influence of the fixed quality, Scorpio characteristics begin to emerge. Combined with the influence of Pluto, these qualities may be manifested positively in your determined, sensitive, passionate, magnetic, and sexually attractive nature. However, the same factors may give you a character that is indifferent, jealous, obsessive, obstinate, and inconsiderate. It is important for you to learn how to show off your positive side. By dressing like a Scorpio you can draw attention to all the good things that make you who you are. If you have a bad reputation by virtue of your zodiac sign, you need to show the world that you never deserved that reputation. You need to look so good that no one will ever have anything bad to say about you again.

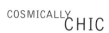
YOUR KEYWORD

As a water sign you have a natural gravity. As a fixed sign you are comfortable are in familiar surroundings. Regardless of your physical size, these characteristics make you a little heavy. You can be compared to a glacier. A glacier is nothing more than frozen water that eventually accumulates into a massive block of ice. Although the glacier may appear to be completely stationary, that is not the case. As it grows it gets heavier, and then it begins to move slowly. By the sheer force of its weight it transforms the landscape around it, carving out a place within its surroundings. *Transformation* is your keyword, Scorpio. Like a glacier, you have the power to transform the world around you. Transformation is important to you because you insist that your environment conform to your standards. Creating a persona that can help you to accomplish this task is within your means. With the power of your mighty zodiac sign, you can carve out your own little niche in the world.

YOUR THREE RULES
TO DRESS BY

1: Sense

Individuals born under a water sign possess a sensate nature. Because they trust their feelings they will regularly judge a situation on the basis of psychic impression rather than reason. Your sign is considered the most psychic of all the signs, and many of you have learned to rely on the sixth sense. You should also trust your senses when you are putting together a wardrobe. Do not allow yourself to get talked into purchasing something you don't feel good in. You'll never wear it, so don't waste your money. When you try on an outfit, you'll sense whether it belongs on you. Even if something looks stunning when you put it on, you need to be sure you get a good feeling from it. Trust your own judgment, Scorpio, because it is uncanny. You'll look better for doing it, and you'll give others a better sense of who you really are.

2: Exert

Scorpios have a remarkable reserve of energy. However, being born under a fixed sign causes many of you to disregard your inherent power. You must learn to exert yourself more forcefully in every aspect of your life—including the manner in which you create your look. You can be one of the best-dressed girls in the zodiac if you endeavor to be, or you can be one of the worst-dressed if you don't put any effort into improving your appearance. Sometimes the fixed quality makes Scorpio women blissfully unaware of how persistently fashion renews itself. You could be dressed in the same style of clothes for years and not realize how foolish you look to the world at large. If this is the case, you need to call upon your reserve of energy. First, force yourself to bring your look up-to-date, then follow up by staying in fashion. By exerting your sense of style vigorously, and making an effort to keep up with the trends, you won't get caught in a look that should have been retired years ago.

3: Transform

Changes in styles can be rather dramatic. A look that was in favor for a few seasons can be abandoned overnight for something completely different. Most women have a difficult time keeping up with the capricious nature of fashion, and Scorpios are no exception. But you also have an extraordinary ability to transform your look. You can walk into a salon and come out looking like a brand-new woman. You can go to the cosmetics counter and walk away virtually unrecognizable as the person you were only moments before. You can overhaul your closet in an afternoon and make it seem like you've purchased an entire new wardrobe. You can take clothing you've grown tired of and alter it in a way that makes you thrilled to wear it again. Pluto has granted you the ability to transform yourself into any kind of woman you want to be. All you have to do is try.

SPECIFICS: WHAT TO WEAR

✧ It is likely that black is very attractive to your sense of style. But the colors that best suit a Scorpio woman are so dark that they could almost be black. Deep red, black-plum, and the most intense midnight blue all look striking on the well-dressed Scorpio.

✧ Although dark colors appeal to you, icy colors look good

on you, too. Frosty blues and greens can go a long way in adding some color to your wardrobe. Silver and white also can brighten up your characteristically dim palette.

✧ When it comes to creating a typical Scorpio look, fabrics are more important than the types of garments you choose. Scorpio women look great in shiny or glossy fabrics. Fluid fabrics that have an icy sheen are especially attractive to you. Sheer fabrics that resemble a layer of frost against your skin can appeal to you as well.

✧ You should try to combine softer fabrics with harder elements. A little hardware looks great on you. For instance, fabrics that are adorned with crystalline beads, sequins, or paillettes may appeal to you. Shark's tooth sequins are especially attractive on a sexy Scorpio woman.

✧ It's likely that you enjoy wearing knitwear. Knit fabrics do suit you, but try to wear knits that are not too chunky and that fit close to your body. As a feminine sign, you are more attractive when you show off your curves.

✧ Softening up your look can help make you more approachable. You have a hard edge to your personality, and many Scorpio women wear clothing that is much too severe. Your gloomy reputation is only made worse when you dress like a funeral director.

✧ Well-tailored clothing suits you better than anything loose. If you do wear loose clothing, it should be made of soft fabrics that move fluidly with your body. Avoid bulky garments at all costs.

✦ The pants you wear should be slim and fitted. The same advice applies to skirts. A slim skirt that ends just below the knee is especially attractive on you. Dresses should fit closely as well, or they should be made from fabrics that cling to your curves.

✦ The structure of close-fitting leather garments is very appealing to your sense of style. A fitted black leather jacket is the quintessential Scorpio garment.

✦ Wearing layered clothing may appeal to you. In fact, layers can help you transform your look at a moment's notice. It may sound like a cliché, but a businesslike jacket worn over a short, sexy dress can take you from day to evening in one simple step.

✦ When you are getting dressed, you must consider the function of the outfit you choose. If you are trying to make yourself more attractive, soften things up. If you are trying to make people take you seriously, let your natural edge shine through. You have the innate power to transform yourself into whoever you want to be, whether that person is as soft as butter or as tough as nails.

✦ You have a passionate nature that endows you with magnetic sex appeal, an essential element of the well-dressed Scorpio woman's wardrobe. In a carefully chosen outfit you can be a hot-blooded vamp or a dangerous femme fatale.

✦ Your sign is associated with the astrological eighth house. This area of a person's chart rules both sex and other people's money. Consequently, many badly dressed Scorpio women look as if they are dressing sexy in order to make money. Unless you're in Hollywood, looking like a streetwalker will never be in style. Learn to exercise good taste when you attempt to dress sexy.

✧ Pluto, your ruling planet, rules over death and the underworld. For this reason, gothic is a characteristic Scorpio style. Wearing one color of clothing exclusively is bad enough, but wearing ugly black clothing exclusively is simply foolish. Don't scare people away with a look that is juvenile and antisocial.

✧ The association of your sign with the occult may affect your wardrobe. As mentioned before, don't dress like a sullen goth or a wanna-be witch. Also avoid dressing like a New Age hippie or an old-world gypsy. There is nothing fashionable about looking like a fool.

✧ An inconsiderate streak can be a Scorpio woman's worst quality. You get wrapped up in your own life far too often, and you sometimes forget about the people who have been there for you when you've needed friends. Your inconsiderate streak can also affect the way you dress by allowing you to believe that your own style is beyond reproach. You could wear a wedding dress to someone else's wedding and not even realize you've done something wrong. It's not arrogance that makes you act inconsiderately but rather indifference to the world around you. Try to be more considerate of others, Scorpio, and always be sure to dress appropriately for the occasion.

WHO TO WEAR

You have a hard edge to your personality that is somewhat responsible for your bad reputation. But a little edge does not make a woman any less beautiful. The designer Helmut Lang knows this. The models at his runway shows typically strut down the catwalk with icy cool looks on their faces. They have tough attitudes that can make them appear emotionless, indifferent, and mysterious. However, the clothing they wear is gorgeous. Despite the apparent edginess of his runway shows, Lang makes clothing that is simple, sexy, and beautiful without ever being prissy. A lot of designer clothing—a Versace dress, for instance—seems sexy on the rack. But Lang's designs seem cold and lifeless on the hangers; they only begin to exude their inherent sex appeal when they are worn. It takes a special kind of woman to pull off Helmut Lang without making herself appear too severe, but you are that kind of woman, Scorpio. You shouldn't allow your chilly demeanor to hide the fact that your blood virtually boils within your veins. Lang makes clothing that helps you reveal a glimpse of the hot-blooded woman lurking behind that cool, expressionless facade.

HELMUT LANG

Don't worry if you can't afford Helmut Lang or other designer clothing. Your talent for transformation allows you to find great clothing in the most unexpected places. It is likely that you have a talent for shopping in secondhand stores.

Whether you scour the racks at the grungiest thrift shops or buy only from the best consignment boutiques, you have a flair for resurrecting outfits that have been passed down by others. You also have the ability to sense the potential in garments that aren't specifically to your liking, and by altering a garment creatively you can transform it into something brand-new. You can even take a vintage outfit that is decades old and wear it like it was hot off the runway. Many people, including many Scorpio women, won't buy previously owned clothing. If that's the case for you, get over this senseless aversion. Swallow your pride, Scorpio. You can have the best wardrobe of any girl in the zodiac if you recognize your innate ability to make what is old new again.

WHAT TO AVOID

There are generally two types of badly dressed Scorpio women. The first is the scary Scorpio woman. Despite the fact that you look great in dark colors and tailored clothing, you must understand that when you look too severe you can frighten people away. Many of you have found that head-to-toe black appeals to you. This is because of your sign's association with the occult. But dressing like a witch can make people think that you are a witch. If you want to scare people away, do it by making them wonder who you had to sell your soul to in order to look so good. Severely tailored clothing can also have a detrimental effect on your public image.

Avoid extreme proportions, like huge shoulder pads. Even though you look great when you are dressed to kill, don't scare everyone away with a look that is as creepy as the animal that gives your sign its name.

The other type of badly dressed Scorpio woman is the sleazy Scorpio woman. She wears tacky, tight clothing that makes the private aspects of her anatomy a matter of public record. She defines her self-image with her sexuality, not realizing that there is much more to looking good than looking lewd. The qualities that make a woman sexy are difficult to pin down. Some people find a woman sexy when she appears to be healthy and energetic. Others may find that a mysterious woman has a great deal of sex appeal. Even more people are attracted to a woman who likes herself: Self-confidence can be the sexiest characteristic of all. All these traits are qualities that you inherit as your astrological birthright, Scorpio. So don't sell yourself short with a look that lets it all hang out.

HAIR AND MAKEUP

Although some women can get away with wearing any hair color, most women are restricted to colors that accentuate their skin tones. Selecting a color that is right for your complexion is important. But regardless of coloring, Scorpio women should wear a hair color that is intense. Jet black hair suits many of you well. You may also look great in a rich, dark brown. Icy white blond may suit you, too. You have an intense personality, and a hair color that is intense complements that characteristic. The style of your hair is also important. As a fixed sign you probably don't change your hairstyle frequently enough; you can get stuck in a rut. However, your innate talent for transforming your appearance ought to make it easy for you to keep up with fashion. But you must make regular appointments at the salon a part of your routine. As far as specific hairstyles are concerned, nothing suits you better than a little mystery. A wave of hair over one of your eyes can make a sexy Scorpio woman like you look drop-dead gorgeous.

Your makeup palette is also dependent on your complexion. But the same rule applies: Intensity becomes you. If you wear cool colors, frosty shades will enhance your look. A little icy blue can be attractive on your eyes. If you wear warm colors, stick to the deepest, darkest reds and plums. The sign of Scorpio rules over reproduction. Scorpio women generally acquire a lovely glow to their skin when they are pregnant. But regardless of your coloring, be sure that you wear mascara and eyeliner. The sexiest Scorpio women always have the most intense "bedroom eyes." If you don't like wearing mascara, consider dyeing your eyelashes a darker color. You may want to darken your eyebrows as well. A glossy sheen looks good on you, too. Avoid matte makeup when the trends allow for it, because a matte finish can give your face a dreary pallor. You are a passionate, hot-blooded woman, and you shouldn't hide behind a mask of dispirited indifference.

ACCESSORIES

Because of your sign's association with sex, Scorpio women generally find that sexy lingerie is an important component of their wardrobes. Black lingerie in particular appeals to your passionate nature. Showing off a little of that lingerie is an ideal way to cultivate some true Scorpio style. If you're wearing a nice bra, let it peek out from beneath a button-front jacket. Or show off a nice camisole underneath a sexy, sheer top. Just be careful that you don't go overboard with the underwear as outerwear look; you'll just end up looking sleazy. Your signature look is more like Victoria's Secret than Frederick's of Hollywood, so try to exercise some good taste when you're showing off your "delicates."

There are many other accessories that appeal to your sense of style. Patent leather shoes and purses suit you perfectly. A pair of glossy black patent leather pumps and a matching handbag are essential elements in your wardrobe. Modern silver jewelry also complements your look, and dramatic pieces can help you add an edge to an otherwise unremarkable outfit. Dark sunglasses may appeal to you, too, and they may help you cultivate that sense of mystery that makes many Scorpio women so desirable. Sexy hosiery also will allow you to make your look more alluring. Fishnet stockings come in and out of fashion on a regular basis. When they're in, you ought to be wearing them, Scorpio—they drive men wild! As with the rest of your wardrobe, try to choose accessories that allow you to look sexy and confident without looking sleazy or scary. Your reputation depends on it.

SOME ADDITIONAL TIPS TO HELP YOU CREATE YOUR OWN COSMIC STYLE

✧ Hide your venomous side behind a sexy floral fragrance.

✧ If you've got a great body, a black bikini is the swimsuit for you.

✧ Remember that "Casual Friday" does not mean "Casual Sex Friday." Unless you are hooker, you shouldn't be dressing like one.

✧ If you are getting married, choose an icy white wedding gown that fits you like a glove. A sequined or beaded bodice will appeal to you. When walking down the aisle, carry a bouquet of exotic, tropical blooms.

✧ A slippery red teddy will appeal to you, and it will probably appeal to anyone else who happens to be in your bedroom.

✧ Paint your nails blood red when you want to look sexy. Wear lipstick to match.

✧ Scorpio women have a tremendous reserve of energy that must be used productively. When you are feeling pent-up, get to the gym and work off some of that excess steam. Your whole look will benefit from your efforts.

✧ As with any of the water signs, your appearance is benefited greatly by water. Drink it. Wash with it. Work out in it.

A FEW WOMEN WHO— FOR BETTER OR WORSE— EXEMPLIFY TRUE SCORPIO STYLE

Hillary Rodham Clinton: October 26

Throughout the trials and tribulations that characterized her reign as First Lady, Hillary Rodham Clinton managed to maintain her icy composure. As a Scorpio, she has a natural talent for making herself appear detached. However, with her humdrum wardrobe she also seemed detached from the world of fashion.

Winona Ryder: October 29

Despite her bad-girl reputation, the actress Winona Ryder is always dressed to kill in typical Scorpio style. She hides her poisonous side well in head-to-toe black, or in the cool, icy colors that complement her sign. But the intensity associated with Scorpio is most evident in her beautiful dark eyes. She is a living illustration of the transformative power of makeup.

Demi Moore: November 11

Demi Moore probably has one of the worst reputations in Hollywood. Despite her numerous achievements (actress, film producer, mother), her reliance upon sex appeal to sell herself has seriously impaired her image. All Scorpio women—including Demi Moore—ought to realize that there's a lot more to looking sexy than letting it all hang out.

Grace Kelly: November 12

The passion that virtually boiled underneath her icy, aristocratic appearance made Grace Kelly a favorite of the film director Alfred Hitchcock. To Hitchcock, it was this mysterious facade that made a woman desirable. Mystery becomes the Scorpio woman.

Whoopi Goldberg: November 13

As a fixed sign, Scorpios must learn that fashion is going to change with them or without them. The comic actress Whoopi Goldberg should learn this, too. Her signature look hasn't changed in years. With her tired old dreadlocks, she appears to have turned her back on all the world of fashion has to offer.

SAGITTARIUS
THE ARCHER

November 22–December 21

WHAT MAKES YOU
A SAGITTARIUS

You've heard it all before, Sagittarius. People say you're fun-loving and adventurous. They tell you you're open-minded and outgoing. They say that you are the life of the party. They may even envy you because they have convinced themselves that being a Sagittarius is delightful. However, if it's so much fun to be born under your sign, then why are so many Sagittarians miserable? How do you explain why you are laughing on the outside and crying on the inside? In general, the reason for this inner suffering is that you feel unfulfilled. You want your life to be fun, but you also want it to be deep and meaningful. When you don't feel as if your life is meaningful, you restlessly stray into controversial situations in an attempt to add meaning to it. Or you wander aimlessly, never really sure of where your misguided existence is going to take you next. Instead of looking into your own heart to discover what would make you happy, you expect to stumble across happiness in your travels. A few of you get lucky and inadvertently discover the so-called meaning of life. However, more of you just go on wandering, hiding your heartache behind a playful laugh and a friendly smile.

The reason you keep smiling is that you possess a genuine sense of optimism. You know that if you keep searching you will eventually discover true happiness. Jupiter, your ruling planet, has endowed you with a very optimistic nature. In Roman mythology Jupiter was the king of the gods. He was blindly optimistic and terribly extravagant. He saw opportunity where it did not always exist, and he was constantly attempting to extricate himself from bad situations. Jupiter has bestowed upon you the same quality. You are quite opportunistic, and, like your mythological ruler, you tend to perceive potential in situations where it does not exist. In addition, you are fiercely independent. However, you can be too independent, and your sense of self-reliance does not always allow you to take good advice when it is offered to you. Like the god Jupiter, you suffer from a lack of discretion: You make a lot of mistakes because of your reckless and carefree nature. This sort of behavior may make you entertaining—you are indeed the life of the party—but it also can get you into a lot of trouble.

Reckless Jupiter isn't the only influence on your sign. Like Aries and Leo, Sagittarius is a fire sign. It is also one of the mutable signs. The fire element adds intuitiveness and physical vigor to your personality. The mutable quality endows you with the ability to see the relevance in any argument. When the extravagant, expansive energy of Jupiter is combined with your fiery, mutable nature, typical Sagittarius characteristics become evident. When these influences are expressed in a positive manner you can be optimistic, fun-loving, nonjudgmental, philosophical, and adventurous. When these influences are expressed negatively you can be irresponsible, gullible, unrealistic, imprudent, and much too opportunistic. Despite your opportunistic temperament, many Sagittarius women are inclined to overlook the opportunities fashion provides. Not only do you fail to keep up with appearances but you also lack the discretion that would allow you to express yourself in an appealing manner. You must realize that looking your best is important because looking good can create opportunities for you. When you dress well—in the style of a Sagittarius—you allow others to see that there is more to your character than just a good time.

YOUR KEYWORD

Control is the keyword you must bear in mind whenever you get dressed. The fire that symbolizes your sign can be compared to a wildfire burning out of control. As it travels the fire gains strength, expanding its range and eventually consuming everything in its path. However, by moving too rapidly the fire can become diffuse and easy to suppress. You, Sagittarius, are like a wildfire because you also have the potential to spread yourself too thinly. In your desire to find yourself, you sometimes wander aimlessly, and like a wildfire you go wherever the wind takes you. Although your ardent, passionate nature endows you with tremendous power, you lose strength by spontaneously changing directions. You must realize that your potency lies in the inherent power of the fire element. You must learn to focus on the task at hand, because it is in your nature to roam. Control must be exercised in all aspects of your life, including your appearance. If you don't learn to use your energy productively, or if you choose to drift through life without any self-restraint, you will burn yourself out. But there is no stopping you if you take the time to apply your energy consistently. Control yourself, Sagittarius, and no one will be able to extinguish the fire that burns within your soul.

YOUR THREE RULES TO DRESS BY

1: Open Your Mind

Fashion offers everyone the opportunity to look better. However, many Sagittarius women view fashion as an oppressive institution. They have bought into the concept that the "fashion system" is harmful to women. The reason they believe this is that men in our society are not required to live up to the same rigorous standards of style and beauty. Whether or not this is true, you must not let it affect the way you dress. Don't allow your idealistic nature to dismiss fashion altogether. You must recognize what the world of fashion has to offer you. As a Sagittarius, you have a very individualistic streak. Why not use fashion to help you personalize your look? You don't have to be trendy to look fashionable. You don't have to be beautiful to look great. But you do have to be aware that fashion is here to stay. Open your mind to fashion, Sagittarius, because looking your best is an opportunity that you would be foolish to ignore.

2: Make It Look Easy

Sagittarius women have a fun-loving nature, and dressing up can be difficult for you. You prefer clothing that is informal to clothing that is dressy. So if the thought of wearing a business suit or a formal dress sends shivers up and down your spine, you must learn to dress suitably. The best-dressed Sagittarian women are able to wear dressy clothing while still appearing comfortable. They choose fabrics and garments that afford them a lot of freedom of movement. They accessorize their outfits to make them look more appropriate for the particular occasion. They have well-maintained hair and makeup that diverts attention away from their rather informal attire. They look put together even when they have put in far less effort than anyone else. Easy, effortless beauty is your look, Sagittarius. Just don't forget that looking like an "effortless beauty" takes a bit of effort.

3: Jump Off the Bandwagon

Many Sagittarius women dislike fashion for philosophical reasons. As mentioned before, many of you dismiss the institution of fashion because you believe that it is oppressive of your gender. You also may regard fashion as artificial, believing that it draws attention away from an individual's character—inner beauty, so to speak. But many women who adopt this position just end up dressing like all of the other women who share the same opinion. They unwittingly jump on the bandwagon. The only difference between these women and trendy women is that they jump on a different bandwagon. A style is a style, regardless of what it is. So if you don't want to look like a poseur, don't adopt an antifashion position and then dress the same as all your friends. Dress to look good, and wear what makes you feel beautiful. The only bandwagon you ever need to jump on is the one you're driving yourself.

SPECIFICS: WHAT TO WEAR

✧ You are very open-minded, Sagittarius. Consequently, the colors you wear are probably a little more adventurous than those most women wear. Members of your sign are unlikely to rely on boring, neutral colors to build up their wardrobes.

✧ The specific colors that suit you well are bright jewel tones. You look great in ruby red, emerald green, sapphire blue, and especially amethyst purple.

✧ Wear any color you want to wear, but try to avoid wearing black on a regular basis. You are the zodiac's most optimistic sign, and wearing too much black can give people the wrong impression of what you're all about.

✧ You can get away with eye-catching mixes of color that make you stand out in a crowd. Wearing loud colors is a typical characteristic of Sagittarian teenagers.

✧ Bold prints and patterns suit you well. In fact, no one wears tartan plaids better than you. Despite their "classic" moniker, tartan plaids are often quite garish. A bright tartan suit jacket is a look that few people can carry off. However, it suits bold Sagittarians ideally.

✧ Your signature look is more downtown than uptown. The best-dressed Sagittarians have a funky, youthful chic, and they never appear haughty or unapproachable.

✧ Well-dressed Sagittarius women are inspired by the world at large. You have an expansive definition of beauty. For this reason you can appropriate the styles of foreign cultures better than anyone else. A season rarely goes by without designers highlighting an ethnic influence in their shows. Open-minded Sagittarius women can easily embrace these styles without appearing to be fashion victims. Try on a sari, a sarong, or a kimono. Put on a dirndl, or some lederhosen. Do whatever makes you feel good—you'll probably start a trend.

✧ You can get away with looking very trendy because people expect you to be trendy. You're a trailblazer by nature, Sagittarius. With your playful sense of style you can inspire others to dress in a more adventurous manner.

✧ You can wear almost any fabric comfortably. However, stretchy, knit fabrics and the high-tech materials of athletic apparel appeal to you more than anything else. It is a priority for you to maintain the ability to move freely and easily in your clothing.

✧ You must control your urge to wear athletic clothing and sporty fabrics where they are not appropriate. You can be a little too carefree, and unwilling to conform to modern standards of etiquette. Dress suitably for the occasion, and don't let people think you're a boor.

✧ Avoid getting into the habit of wearing fabrics and styles that are outdoorsy. The look of Eddie Bauer may appeal to you, but you shouldn't live in clothes like that.

✧ Remember that you can't be the life of the party without a party dress or two in your closet.

✧ The specific garments that appeal to you provide you with a sense of freedom. For this reason it is likely that you wear pants often. Jeans and other casual styles suit you well. Sagittarians are particularly fond of stretchy pants.

✧ Sagittarius rules over the thighs, causing many of you

Sagittarius women to be hypersensitive about the size of their thighs. Although you generally prefer pants, skirts are usually more forgiving than pants when it comes to large legs. Don't draw undue attention to your thighs, and perhaps your "problem area" will seem less problematic.

✧ Many larger Sagittarius women tend to hide behind baggy clothes. Dressing in oversized garments will not make you look slimmer. Control the urge to run away from yourself. Learn to love your body, or do whatever is necessary to change your shape until you love your body. You have energy to burn, Sagittarius, so burn some off at the gym. You'll look and feel better.

✧ Avoid superfluous fabric and excessive layering. Don't bulk up your silhouette by putting on too many things at once.

✧ Certain looks from the past appeal to you. You are especially fond of the eras when fashion changed drastically. The hippie look that characterized the late 1960s is a classic Sagittarius style. However, it was in fashion decades ago. Too many poorly dressed Sagittarians are still wearing the same old "granola" look today. Many of them also believe that they are still on the cutting edge in their antifashion look. Nothing could be further from the truth.

WHO TO WEAR

The designer whose clothing best exemplifies the positive qualities of your sign is Vivienne Tam. From a business standpoint, she may not be in the same league as designers like Karl Lagerfeld or Calvin Klein. However, she is definitely in the same league artistically. Vivienne Tam is brilliant, and her ability to create beautiful clothing is indisputable. She derives inspiration for her collections from foreign lands and popular culture. However, there is nothing derivative about the clothing she makes. She is a modern artist, like Picasso or Matisse, who seeks enlightenment from the world around her in order to create something altogether new. Her Chairman Mao dress is one of the most modern and influential garments of the twentieth century. But unlike many of the fashion world's artists, Tam creates completely wearable clothing. She prefers contemporary fabrics that allow the wearer to move without restraint. There is a sportswearlike feel to her apparel that appeals to your casual nature. In Tam's signature designs, a woman like you can look comfortable, fashionable, artistic, philosophical, open-minded, and beautiful all at once. Could it get any better than that, Sagittarius?

Vivienne Tam

Many other labels suit you well. The Italian label Moschino may appeal to you because of the playful, tongue-in-cheek manner in which it pokes fun at the fashion system. Because you also find athletic clothing appealing, you likely have something by Nike in your closet. Despite all the competition, Nike still manages to produce some of the most funky, fashionable athletic apparel on the market. Just don't live in athletic clothing, Sagittarius—even if you are an athlete. Jeans wear lines probably appeal to you, too. However, you are quite an individual, so you probably shun the more popular brands. For instance, if you had to make a choice between Diesel and Tommy Hilfiger, you would undoubtedly choose Diesel, simply because it's less common. Clothing in this price range also appeals to you, because you normally don't spend a lot on clothing. And you shouldn't. You quickly grow tired of your clothes, in much the way you grow tired of being in the same place for too long.

WHAT TO AVOID

Many poorly dressed Sagittarius women don't appreciate fashion at all. They dress in whatever they grab. Their hair is a mess because they can't be bothered to do anything with it. They wear no makeup because they own no makeup. In an attempt to make a philosophical statement about the importance of individual character, they disregard their looks entirely. They preach the evils of the modern "fashion system," yet they neglect to realize that fashion is hardly modern: Thousands of years ago the ancient Egyptians had ideals of beauty that make our modern standards pale in comparison. Sagittarians stress the idea that beauty is only skin deep while disregarding the scientific evidence that explains how certain standards of beauty are a result of evolution, not social conditioning. They are idealists, and their misguided idealism makes them think looks don't matter. Consequently, they look awful.

Another type of badly dressed Sagittarian woman is the excessive woman. The excessive woman does not exercise any self-control. She may be a clotheshorse who cannot stop herself from buying designer outfits. She may go overboard with the makeup and end up looking like a clown. Or she might be a tacky mess who insists that every inch of her outfit should be covered in rhinestones. She looks bad because she has not learned when to say no to herself. All of you must realize that having Jupiter as your ruling planet can make you a little too eager. Sometimes you need to temper your enthusiasm, because you can see opportunities where they do not exist. If one designer outfit looks good on you, you won't necessarily look better if you buy the whole line. If a little color makes your complexion look nice, a lot of color won't always make you look better. You can have too much of a good thing, Sagittarius. Exercise some discretion, and learn to control your enthusiasm. Your whole look depends on it.

HAIR AND MAKEUP

Effortless beauty is your look, Sagittarius. However, the term "effortless beauty" does not mean that you are guaranteed to look beautiful without putting in any effort. More accurately, it means looking beautiful without looking artificial. The secret to cultivating this look begins with your skin-care regimen. You must put in the effort required to have a naturally beautiful complexion. For some of you that entails nothing more than washing with soap and water. For others it can mean regular visits to a dermatologist. Flawless skin becomes you. Therefore, it is the foundation of your look. As far as cosmetics are concerned, you look your best when you wear light, fresh makeup. Your adventurous nature makes you receptive to new trends, so you should have no problem wearing fashionable colors in a modern manner. Just remember to strike a balance between your nonchalant nature and your tendency toward excess, or all of your effort will be wasted on a look that just isn't your style.

Your hairstyle also needs to tread the fine line between nonchalance and excess. A good haircut will allow you to do this. You probably don't like to primp in front of the mirror, and you probably dislike using a lot of styling products in your hair. There's nothing wrong with that. However, many of you fail to maintain your hairstyles. You get a great cut that you wear well, but then you let it grow out too long. The result is a sloppy, unkempt mop. Regular appointments with a hairstylist must be part of your routine. If it's been months since you've been to a salon, then it is time to go back. Be frank with the stylist, and let him or her know that you don't spend a lot of time on your hair. Insist upon a cut that will allow you to cultivate the effortless beauty that suits you so well. Also, remember that shorter hair is easier to maintain. A trendy, sporty cut could make your beauty regimen—and your life—much less complicated.

ACCESSORIES

Of all the women in the zodiac, Sagittarians are the most likely to eschew purses. You dislike old-style bags, and you favor carrying nothing over carrying something that just isn't you. But instead of shoving everything you need into your overstuffed pockets, you should find a bag that suits your casual lifestyle. There are many modern, sporty bags on the market that are no bigger than a large wallet. You probably don't need a large bag, because you generally don't carry your entire collection of cosmetics in your purse. A small purse in an untraditional fabric or a high-tech synthetic material will suit you much better than a classic handbag from one of the prestige lines. Kate Spade makes marvelous, funky bags that appeal to your "downtown" sense of style. Even if you have a style that demands a more classic look, you are likely to prefer modern. Just be careful to choose something that is appropriate for the outfit you are wearing. Wearing a knapsack with a cocktail dress can be rather gauche.

Most Sagittarius women don't wear high heels unless they have to. You prefer casual shoes to dressier styles, and you likely have a fondness for rubber-soled shoes. Just be careful to avoid putting on athletic shoes with every outfit you wear.

Accessories usually don't play an important part in the way you dress. Many of you barely bother to dress up at all, so adding accessories to an outfit is rarely your priority. But well-chosen accessories can be the cornerstone of your wardrobe, Sagittarius. You prefer informal garments to anything formal or restrictive of your movement. By utilizing accessories you can make yourself look more "put together" than you actually are. Ethnic jewelry suits your sense of style well. You may find turquoise especially attractive. Carefully chosen scarves, hats, jewelry, eyewear, leg wear, and shoes can allow you to make your own look less nonchalant and more befitting of the occasion. If you call upon your innate resourcefulness, you can look stylish in the simplest outfits without compromising your comfort level. Learn to use accessories wisely, Sagittarius, and you'll discover that you can possess a great wardrobe without ever having to dress yourself up.

SOME ADDITIONAL TIPS TO HELP YOU CREATE YOUR OWN COSMIC STYLE

✧ A lively, fresh fragrance will suit you well. A subtle hint of exotic spice or fragrant wood in your perfume will appeal to you, too.

✧ Remember that "Casual Friday" does not give you the license to dress like a slob.

✧ If you are planning a wedding, get married in something short and untraditional. You'll feel great in a cocktail-length dress. Carry a bouquet of gorgeous red tulips down the aisle.

✧ The classic cut of an athletic swimsuit will appeal to your sporty nature.

✧ Sporty undergarments suit you well, but keep an open mind when it comes to lingerie in general. Most Sagittarius women are unaware of their own sex appeal.

✧ Outer beauty is often a reflection of your vitality. Your whole look suffers when you are inactive.

✧ Many Sagittarians underestimate the value of a good night's sleep.

✧ Nicely manicured hands can help you pull your look together. Even if you keep your nails short, paint them a trendy color.

✧ You probably wear a sloppy, oversized T-shirt to bed. There's nothing wrong with that, unless you're trying to impress the person beside you.

A FEW WOMEN WHO — FOR BETTER OR WORSE — EXEMPLIFY TRUE SAGITTARIUS STYLE

Tina Turner: November 26

Most celebrities who have spent decades in the spotlight have very individualistic styles. Tina Turner is no exception. With her wild hairstyle she is one of the most recognizable women in the world. Like any well-dressed Sagittarian, she knows how to be herself while still looking beautiful to everyone else.

Bette Midler: December 1

Early in her career Bette Midler realized that her biggest talent was her individuality. Beyond her prowess as an entertainer, people love to see her because they love her personality. Because she dresses like a true individual, her character is able to shine through every outfit she wears.

Tyra Banks: December 4

Tyra Banks exemplifies all that is wonderful about the well-dressed Sagittarius woman. In youthful, adventurous outfits and modern makeup, she is one of the world's most desirable women. With her fun-loving, effortless style, she makes looking good look easy.

Sinéad O'Connor: December 8

Sagittarians are trailblazers by nature. In the late 1980s the songbird Sinéad O'Connor shaved her head and started a trend. In typical Sagittarius style she challenged the ideals of beauty in a decade characterized by big hair. Whether or not she was aware of what she had started, her idealistic stance made her a fashion icon.

Florence Griffith Joyner: December 21

The world has never known a woman quite like Florence
Griffith Joyner. Being the world's best female athlete just
wasn't enough for Flo-Jo—she had to show exactly who she
was. With her one-of-a-kind tracksuits and her ridiculously
painted fingernails, she was the personification of Sagittarian
individuality.

CAPRICORN
THE SEA GOAT

December 22–January 19

WHAT MAKES YOU A CAPRICORN

Capricorn, you are a bore—or at least that's what everyone tells you. They say you're too serious. They tell you you're too traditional. They envy your businesslike virtues, yet they condemn the coldhearted way you conduct your business. Even worse, they treat you as if you have no personality. This is not an accurate description. They neglect to observe that a human being exists behind that composed facade. You've simply been a victim of bad public relations. You know you're not too serious: If you were that serious you wouldn't have the best

sense of humor in the zodiac. You know you're not too traditional: If you were that traditional you wouldn't be so great
at reinventing trends. You also know how many times you've
had to hit rock bottom before you've had any success.
Nevertheless, there is a reason people don't understand you.
It's because you are aloof, and you don't really care whether
they understand you. You do not suffer fools gladly, and you're
too practical to waste your time explaining yourself to people
who cannot comprehend what you're trying to say. In fact,
you rarely waste your time at all. Precious time is the only
commodity that Capricorns truly value.

Capricorn is ruled by Saturn, the so-called timekeeper of
the zodiac. Saturn endows the members of your sign with
impeccable timing. You have a brilliant, witty sense of humor
that depends on good timing. You also have the ability to look
back into the past to anticipate what will happen in the
future. There's nothing psychic about the way you foresee the
future—you just apprehend the cyclical nature of things. You
notice when the circumstances around you bear similarities
to events that have occurred before. As you age you learn to
expect the repetition of these cycles, and you begin to
develop a sense of caution that seldom allows you to repeat
your mistakes. Consequently, your life seems to get better
and better as you grow older. However, along with good timing, Saturn imparts to you a sense of gravity that can make
you seem quite dull. Saturn can be like a wet blanket on your
personality, endowing you with a heavy demeanor that others

view as threatening and unattractive. Depending on how you deal with the influence of your ruling planet, Saturn can either help or hinder your progress. It's not an easy situation to be in, Capricorn.

In addition to the mixed influences of Saturn, Capricorn is one of the earth signs. It is also one of the cardinal signs. Your innate self-assurance can be attributed to the cardinal quality: People born under a cardinal sign generally don't waste time making a decision. The earth element provides your material nature. You thrive on the comforts the physical world provides. When this earthy temperament is combined with cardinal confidence, Capricorn character traits begin to appear. Together with the influence of Saturn, these factors give rise to typical Capricorn qualities. Expressed in a positive manner these qualities include self-discipline, perseverance, patience, great ambition, and common sense. Expressed in a negative manner they include arrogance, obstinacy, cynicism, frugality, and a manipulative nature. It is no wonder people speak badly of you when you exhibit those negative qualities. Your public image only gets worse when you dress in a severe manner. You enjoy being complimented on your appearance. However, try to be humble when you are complimented. You can be a snob. You need to practice some public relations of your own, Capricorn. You are not the serious, coldhearted snake your critics have made you out to be. If you take the time to draw attention to your positive qualities, you can show everyone that there is good side to your

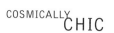
character. Start dressing in the style of your sign, and let the world know how seriously remarkable you are.

YOUR KEYWORD

The keyword you must remember when getting dressed is *stature*. Picture the earth that symbolizes your sign as the earth that builds mountains. Mountains are created when the tectonic plates that make up the earth's crust collide. As these massive sheets slowly push against one another, they are forced upward, creating giant outcrops of rock that dominate the landscape. You, Capricorn, are like a mountain because you also have a tendency to dominate the scene. You persistently force your way into a situation, gradually and imperceptibly advancing until you ultimately assume the "stature" you desire. However, this does not happen overnight. It is a slow, uphill battle for you. From time to time you move forward too quickly, causing all your hard work to crash down around you like an avalanche. But you take these setbacks in stride, and you learn from your mistakes. Along the way you develop patience, and an appreciation for the magnitude of your accomplishments. In time you rebuild the solid base that inevitably allows you to achieve the stature you seek. And at the end, Capricorn, you virtually tower over the world around you.

YOUR THREE RULES TO DRESS BY

1: Buy

You have a methodical way of doing things that is well-suited to the world of big business. That quality may make you rich. The same quality can make you look like a million bucks. The well-dressed Capricorn woman knows that building a wardrobe successfully is a time-consuming enterprise. She systematically acquires the items that will make her wardrobe exceptional. She shops persistently to ensure that everything in her closet allows her to stay one step ahead of the competition. She routinely buys beautiful clothing, because she knows that looking good is an investment in her future. Unfortunately, too few Capricorn women have such orderly shopping habits. Many of you are frugal, and you refuse to spend money on anything you believe is frivolous, like fashion. But spending money on clothing that makes you look good is important. Looking good gives you a competitive edge, because when you look good people treat you better. It may not be fair, Capricorn, but it's the way of the world. Don't ever undervalue the power of beauty.

2: Sell

Not only do you need to buy a look that flatters you but you also need to know how to sell that look. So remember this,

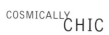

Capricorn: Sex sells. Using sex to sell your look can be easy for you. The earth element endows you with a palpable sex appeal. You're no fantasy girl—you're the real thing. Consequently, playing up your earthy sensuality is an essential element of true Capricorn style. Your reserved bearing makes you appear seductive yet unattainable, and people often desire what they cannot have. Don't worry if you feel as though you are appealing to the lowest common denominator by dressing seductively—you won't be the first person to try it. Wear your clothes a little tighter. Wear your dresses a little shorter. Wear your heels a little higher. Show a little skin with an open-collar blouse or a high-slit skirt. Just remember that an understated approach to dressing sexy suits you better than an overtly sleazy look. A subtle, seductive look becomes you, Capricorn. It's in the stars.

3: Have Fun

You were born under the wittiest sign of the zodiac. You have a wry sense of humor that goes over the heads of an unrefined audience—some people just don't get you. Your jokes are sophisticated, well-timed, and always a little inappropriate. Your witty nature also affects the way you dress. More than any other sign, Capricorns can get away with kitsch. You can put on an outfit that is ridiculously outdated, yet still make it look stylish. You can do something silly with your hair, then walk around as if nothing has changed. You can dress up in a gorilla suit and perform a little song and dance, like Marlene Dietrich in *Blonde Venus* (1932). The reason you can act foolishly without looking like a fool is that you intimidate people. No one is going to tell someone with an ego as big as yours that she looks absurd. So have some fun with fashion. Play around and show off your lighter side every now and then. The people who "get" you will appreciate the entertainment.

SPECIFICS: WHAT TO WEAR

✧ Black is your color, Capricorn. Many women wear black exclusively because they believe that wearing just one color will simplify their wardrobes. But you shouldn't wear black because it makes your life simple; you should wear it because it makes you look hot.

✧ Dark colors generally appeal to you more than anything bright. Although a little soft gray or icy mauve may make its way into your closet, you are definitely not a pastel person.

✧ The secret to wearing black successfully without looking somber is this: Show off just enough skin so that no one notices the color you're wearing.

✧ You can get away with wearing apparel that is sexier than what most women wear, but the things you look the sexiest in are never trashy. In fact, they are usually quite simple. For instance, you look great in a tailored white dress shirt when you undo too many buttons.

✧ Avoid prissy details like peplums or leg-of-mutton sleeves on your clothes. Also, avoid fluffy fibers, like mohair or angora. Cute is a style you'll never pull off.

✧ The fabrics that suit you the best are simple. Even when you wear luxury fabrics, you likely shun complex materials, like brocade or lace.

✧ You rarely wear prints or patterns. However, your sense of humor allows you to appreciate the comic value of certain prints. For instance, wearing something like a zebra-printed dress for a special occasion could put a smile on your face. Try it for yourself.

✧ If your business attire seems drab, jazz it up with some patterned garments. Houndstooth, glen plaid, and other classic patterns appeal to your practical nature.

✧ You look great in business clothes. Try to wear more suits, straight-legged pants, fitted skirts, and well-tailored jackets.

✧ Capricorn rules the knees. Many Capricorn women have gorgeous legs that look great in skirts cut just above the knee.

✧ Your innate sex appeal allows you to look good in tight clothes—even in something as understated as a tight pair of Levi's 501s.

✧ Many Capricorns are exceptionally body-conscious. You treat your body like a status symbol. When you have a great body, you like to show it off in stretchy, high-tech athletic fabrics.

✧ Capricorn women love black leather. Leather has an earthy, sensual appeal that many of you find irresistible. You even like the smell of leather.

✧ Aside from being the ideal choice for your shoes, belts,

and other accessories, leather can play an integral role in your wardrobe. However, you need to choose garments that are sexy rather than tacky. Even though you would probably look good in a studded leather bra, biker chic is hardly your style.

✧ Glossy fabrics that have a leatherlike sheen look great on you. A black dress in a satiny fabric is an essential addition to your wardrobe. The classic little black dress is the quintessential Capricorn garment.

✧ Many of you are very status conscious. You like to wear designer labels because you believe they afford you prestige. However, the way you wear your clothes can give you stature regardless of what you're wearing. The best-dressed Capricorn women have a natural air of prestige.

✧ The influence of Saturn can affect the way you dress. Saturn gives you a profound appreciation for the past, so you can wear vintage clothing well. Keep your eyes open and you may find something valuable, like a vintage couture dress, in a consignment boutique.

✧ Even though most of you are not bargain hunters, Capricorns generally stumble across good deals without having to rummage through sales racks or outlet malls. The reason for this is that you know the value of things. You rarely buy clothes just because they're inexpensive. You buy them because you want them.

✧ You are well-mannered, and you usually dress appropriately for the occasion. However, some of you have a

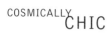

difficult time dressing down. Learn to cut loose every now and then, Capricorn.

WHO TO WEAR

There is no designer label that suits your Capricorn style better than Tom Ford for Gucci. The Gucci label has always been a status symbol. But when Tom Ford took over

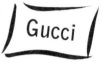

design duties at the house of Gucci, he brought sex appeal back to a label that had not been sexy for years. Without compromising the luxurious image of Gucci, he reinvented the company and turned it into one of the world's most fashionable brands. Although his clothes are cut rather classically, Ford executes his designs in a way that makes the wearer look seductive. He uses fabrics that cling in just the right places. He slits skirts in a manner that is sexy without being lurid. He molds leather jackets until they fit like a second skin. He takes inspiration from the past and makes it look brand-new. He is also witty. His designs often poke fun at retro styles, but in a manner that pays homage to the looks rather than demeaning them. With Tom Ford at the creative helm of Gucci, the label exemplifies wit, sex appeal, and prestige—in other words, everything that is wonderful about the well-dressed Capricorn woman.

Even if you can't afford Gucci, you should have no problem finding outfits that suit your sense of style. Tom Ford's sexy designs are knocked off routinely by other apparel manufacturers. But if you don't feel comfortable dressing in a sexy manner, there are plenty of other labels you can turn to. Several of the finer department stores carry house labels that appeal to the conservative, businesslike side of your character. If you lead a life that allows you to wear more informal clothing, much of Banana Republic's casual wear will appeal to your earthy nature. You also look great in simple, classic garments, like a pair of jeans. Just be sure to wear a fitted, figure-flattering style. You're lucky, Capricorn, because underneath that aloof attitude is a very sensible girl. You're so practical that you'll always be able to find something that looks good on you.

WHAT TO AVOID

The worst-dressed Capricorn woman is unstylish. She feels the dreary influence of Saturn acutely. Consequently, her ruling planet throws a wet blanket on her personality as well as her sense of style. She wears clothing that is grave and far too conservative. Because she takes herself too seriously, she projects an image that others view as dull and unimaginative. Relying upon the strength of her character to define her persona, she neglects to realize that she lives in a very superficial world. If you are one of these unstylish Capricorn women, you must understand that looks and style do matter, and that they will continue to matter as long as people value beauty. A woman with a beautiful garden is not considered superficial just because she chooses to beautify her surroundings. So why do so many people consider a woman superficial because she attempts to make herself as beautiful as possible? Don't let yourself get confused by this double standard, Capricorn. Worry about pleasing yourself, and find a personal style that makes you feel happy about the way you look.

Something else that Capricorns should avoid is materialism. Capricorn is considered the most materialistic sign in the zodiac—you like the things money can buy. But there is another side to this materialistic nature that has little to do with wealth. Sometimes Capricorns find themselves interested solely in the physical aspects of life. They are greedy. They eat too much, drink too much, smoke too much, wear too much, have too much sex, and so on. Despite their inherent self-discipline, they consume everything in their paths. You must learn that there is more to life than what is tangible: your inner beauty, for instance. The way you feel on the inside is reflected in the way you look on the outside. Learn to recognize the connection between how you feel and how you look, and you will allow others to see that there is more to your personality than what meets the eye.

HAIR AND MAKEUP

You are not the trendiest sign of the zodiac, Capricorn. You normally don't buy into trends because you have the common sense to realize that most styles are short-lived. Therefore, you ought to wear your hair in a style that is not terribly trendy. You also should avoid hairdos that make you appear haughty. A simple cut that shows off a healthy head of hair is more attractive on you than an overprocessed helmet of country club hair. So take care of your hair. You likely have a healthy complexion that is enhanced by a warm, earthy hair color. Unless you're trying to cultivate a more severe look, avoid severe colors, like blue-black or platinum blond. Also, don't do anything cute with your hair. Most of you Capricorn girls grew out of pigtails before you could tie your own.

You tend to shop at the finest cosmetics counters. Your makeup is carefully chosen and remarkably tasteful. But you do have a dirty little secret. Despite your desire to dominate the scene socially by obtaining status symbols and acting aloof, you are a pragmatist at heart. Somewhere in your makeup bag, underneath the Estée Lauder compact and those Dior lipsticks, is something like an inexpensive tube of Maybelline Great Lash mascara. You know a good product when you see it. However, you may be a little too haughty to use it when anyone's looking your way. You probably wash your face with simple, inexpensive soap, too. Capricorn women rarely spend a lot of money on skin-care products. As you grow older it becomes apparent to you that your skin condition reflects on your overall vitality. You begin to notice that you look bad when you're stressed out, so you take evasive action and practice adequate stress reduction—exercise, for instance. Practical solutions to problems like this allow you to remain young looking while everyone around you withers away. You like that, Capricorn. Nothing pleases you more than winning at the end. Note that if your complexion allows, you should stick to earthy colors when choosing cosmetics. Wear deep plums and earthy reds instead of pinks and peaches.

ACCESSORIES

As status-conscious as you are, it is unlikely that you walk around dripping with diamonds. You like to show off, but you have a very understated manner. You like to wear jewelry, but only if it is worth wearing. You're too snobby to wear most costume jewelry. If everything you owned came from Harry Winston, you would probably make an effort to wear it more often. A Capricorn woman usually prefers to show off with a gorgeous designer purse. Strutting around nonchalantly with a fabulous Gucci bag hanging from your shoulder is more your style. You normally carry a black purse, since it matches all the black clothing you wear. You should try to stick to black exclusively when you purchase handbags, shoes, belts, and other accessories. Carry a black wallet as well. You are a material girl, and a gorgeous wallet can make you feel like you're rich even when that wallet is empty. A gorgeous watch from a prestigious line like Cartier is the ultimate Capricorn accessory. You value fine timepieces as much as you value time itself.

Take care when purchasing other accessories. Using accessories to modernize is a cost-effective way to revitalize your wardrobe. But poorly chosen accessories can cheapen up an outfit just as easily. You are not a cheap woman, and you are certainly not a cheap-looking woman. So wear only the best when it comes to accessories. Your hosiery is especially important. Choose hosiery that is sexy and well-made. Whenever the current trends allow, wear styles that have texture. Lacy styles, fine fishnets, or other patterns suit you well. Black hosiery appeals to you, and nude hosiery looks great on you, too. But the most important factor to remember when purchasing hosiery is fabric weight: You look your best in sheer styles. Many of you have gorgeous legs, and opaque hosiery does not do you justice. If dark legs are in style, Capricorn, maybe you should be wearing pants.

SOME ADDITIONAL TIPS TO HELP YOU CREATE YOUR OWN COSMIC STYLE

✧ Many of you like black so much that you paint your fingernails black. Try not to make this a habit. Keep your look versatile by wearing a wide variety of colors. Gold, platinum, and other metallic colors also work well for you.

✧ Floral fragrances with a hint of greenery appeal to your earthy nature.

✧ A formal wedding dress will suit you when you walk down the aisle. Avoid impractical details, like a long train on your gown. Carry a bouquet of gorgeous white lilies.

- ✧ Sexy black lingerie appeals to you. But you're practical, so you probably wear ordinary cotton panties.
- ✧ Some of you can be so status-conscious that you insist on wearing designer labels in places where hardly anyone sees them, including your bed.
- ✧ If you're daring, show off some skin at the beach in a tiny black bikini.
- ✧ Capricorn rules the joints, particularly the knees. Many Capricorn women have strong knees. For this reason, jogging may appeal to you. If you are a jogger, do your joints a favor and wear quality footwear designed specifically for jogging.
- ✧ Use "Casual Friday" to show that you are not the excessively serious woman people think you are. Shock everyone in the office by wearing a color to work—and not navy blue!

A FEW WOMEN WHO— FOR BETTER OR WORSE— EXEMPLIFY TRUE CAPRICORN STYLE

Annie Lennox: December 25

The pop diva Annie Lennox has one of the best faces the world has ever seen. No one wears makeup better. But behind that makeup is a mature woman whose talent seems to grow more exceptional as she ages. Like the typical Capricorn woman, she just gets better and better.

Marlene Dietrich: December 27

The Capricorn actress Marlene Dietrich had a one-of-a-kind look that made her a screen legend. However, what gave her true cosmic chic was how aloof she appeared. With a simple glance from behind those long eyelashes, she could make anyone feel a little bit smaller.

Gabrielle Reece: January 6

Capricorns like to have it all. Not only is gorgeous Gabrielle Reece an Olympic athlete but she's also a highly paid model. With her strong sense of self-discipline, and abdominal muscles most women would kill for, she has made it to the top of the mountain in typical Capricorn style.

Kate Moss: January 16

Kate Moss made herself a career in a business where she is an anomaly. She is too short to be a model, and she doesn't even look like a model. But she is a consummate professional, and her body of work speaks for itself. In characteristic Capricorn style she works hard, and she reaps the rewards of her hard work unrepentantly.

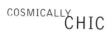
Dolly Parton: January 19

Capricorns are better than anyone else at marketing their own image. Dolly Parton has done exactly that. Like her fellow Capricorn Elvis Presley, Dolly has turned herself into a tourist attraction. While she may not appear fashionable to her harshest critics, like any good Capricorn girl she's laughing all the way to the bank.

ELEVEN

AQUARIUS
THE WATER BEARER

January 20–February 18

WHAT MAKES YOU
AN AQUARIUS

Of all the zodiac signs, Aquarians seem to be the most difficult to understand. The reason for this is the position of the sun in your chart. When the sun is in Aquarius it is at its weakest point— what astrologers call its detriment. Because of your weak sun sign, it is likely that other factors in your chart have a dominant effect on your personality. So your horoscope hardly ever offers profound insight into your future. For this reason most Aquarians are skeptical of astrology. However, there is nothing wrong with astrology itself. The real problem is that it is not meant to work in the manner you expect it to. Your sun sign isn't supposed to be a window into the future. More accurately, the sun rules your self-expression. Fashion is also concerned with self-expression. Whether or not you demonstrate all the typical characteristics of your sign, you can benefit by expressing yourself in an essentially Aquarian style.

Uranus is your ruling planet, and it imparts to all Aquarians an extremely individualistic streak. You are the zodiac's true eccentrics. Even if you are very conservative, you likely have a quirky personality. These idiosyncrasies are ingrained in your character, although they may surface only occasionally. When you do reveal your Aquarian side, it is often in flashes of creative brilliance or wildly unpredictable behavior. Your unpredictability may be one of the reasons astrologers have such a difficult time characterizing you. You're also rather erratic. This is because slow-moving Uranus takes about seven years to progress through a single zodiac sign. When it does make a move from one sign to the next, your priorities undergo an upheaval. This "seven-year itch" causes you to reevaluate your life, and it often results in drastic changes to the way you think. If there is just one thing all Aquarians have in common, it is the way you think. Your thought process evolves unceasingly, and what you believe is important to you on one day may be inconsequential on the next. Uranus thrives on these changes. Consequently, Aquarians were born to change.

Unfortunately, some of you don't like to change. Aquarius is one of the fixed signs. Individuals born under a fixed sign often have a difficult time accepting that change is inevitable. Because of this, many Aquarians can get stuck in a bad situation for years. When you finally attempt to extricate yourself, you tend to do it suddenly and unexpectedly. The unstable influence of Uranus is quite incompatible with the steadfast nature of the fixed quality. However, Aquarius is also an air sign, along with Gemini and Libra. The air element endows you with reason. Your rational thought process allows you to understand your erratic behavior. When all these factors are combined, typical Aquarian characteristics emerge. On the positive side you can be independent, original, intellectual, sociable, and kindhearted. On the negative side you can be perverse, unpredictable, emotionally detached, disagreeable, and rebellious. Regardless of the fact that astrology has let you down in the past, you should try to express your positive Aquarian qualities. By doing so you will let people know you a little better. You must strive to be the best Aquarius that you can be. Dressing in an Aquarian style will allow you to show the world your best side. You need to let everyone know that it takes more than a weak sun sign to keep you from looking like the most gorgeous girl in the zodiac.

YOUR KEYWORD

The keyword that most appropriately defines the well-dressed Aquarius woman is *electricity*. The air that symbolizes your sign can be compared to a neon light. Neon is a colorless gas, and it is indistinguishable from the rest of the elements that make up the air. But when a current of electricity is passed through neon, it shines brilliantly. You are like neon because you also have the potential to shine. You have a dazzling personality that can go unnoticed because you fail to recognize just how spectacular you can be. You often express the colorless aspects of your character while disregarding the brilliant quirks that make you such a unique individual. Instead of allowing your eccentricities to electrify your appearance, you simply float around, unappreciated and overlooked. You must learn to express yourself in an electric manner: one that is both radiant and exciting. By adopting a more exciting style of dress, you can light up the world around you.

YOUR THREE RULES TO DRESS BY

1: Express

As mentioned before, the sun rules your sense of self-expression. With your weak sun sign, many have a difficult time expressing your individuality. You know that there is much more to your personality than what meets the eye, but you don't know how to express it without drawing undue attention to yourself. Therein lies your problem, Aquarius. You are the most original, unpredictable individual in the zodiac, so why would you even try to blend in? Dressing in a mediocre style defies your character: You were born to be fabulous. You can turn heads. You can buck trends. You can shock the world with a look that is absolutely unique. By dressing in an essentially Aquarian manner, you can express the unconventional aspects of your personality rather than concealing your quirks behind a commonplace mask. Don't even try to fit in, Aquarius. Just be who you want to be.

2: Modernize

No other zodiac sign embraces the future more willingly than yours, Aquarius. Generally, Aquarians are the first people to own the latest in technological gadgetry. Uranus endows you with a fondness for the modern. Many of you work in high-tech or scientific occupations, and some of you are great fans of futuristic science fiction. Moreover, many of the best-dressed Aquarius women have a bold, modern style. A great deal of what fashion designers create is retro, and truly modern looks are an anomaly in a business often obsessed with nostalgia. For this reason a woman who dresses in futuristic apparel can appear to be unique. Why not cultivate a personal style that allows you to express your distinctiveness? Modernize your wardrobe, Aquarius, and you can create a future in which no one looks better than you.

3: Shock

Some astrologers have described the wavy lines that represent your sign as waves of electricity. This is an apt description because there is a shockingly electric air to many well-dressed

Aquarius women. However, the electricity that defines these women is not generated from shock value. Instead, it is created quite subtly. The best-dressed Aquarius woman invents a look that expresses the individual aspects of her personality. She may have a rather bohemian way of dressing, or she may appear uncommonly glamorous. But she is unquestionably distinct. In a world where most people attempt to imitate the personal styles of others, there is something truly shocking about dressing in an individual manner. All of you have an unconventional streak that should not go unrecognized. You need to express your eccentricity. You can shock the world just by being yourself.

SPECIFICS: WHAT TO WEAR

✧ Electric blue is generally considered the quintessential Aquarius color. Other electric colors appeal to you, too. Neonlike brights are especially attractive to a bold Aquarius woman.

✧ Silver, copper, and titanium suit you well. Bright white also looks great on you.

✧ Many of you love black. You can get away with black as long as you wear it in a manner that is not colorless. If you choose to wear black on a regular basis, be sure the garments you wear are unique; otherwise you'll just blend into the background.

✧ The specific garments you wear well are just as individual as your character. However, you should avoid wearing pants exclusively. Because Aquarius is a fixed sign, many of you get far too comfortable doing the same thing over and over again. For this reason, you could spend your entire life in tired blue jeans or boring khakis.

✧ Each zodiac sign rules over a particular region of the body. For Aquarians that region is the lower leg. You look good in cropped pants and in other styles that draw attention to this area. You should also wear skirts that show off your calves. Wear a sexy anklet, too.

✧ You should never attempt to wear the fashionable skirt length. Wear what looks good on you, and what looks good with the rest of your outfit.

✧ Pants made of light, breezy materials suit you better than those made from stiff fabrics. Even though you were born in the middle of winter, summery fabrics look great on you.

✧ You often purchase an outfit because it has odd details that you find appealing.

✧ Clothes that are designed with unusual proportions are especially attractive on you.

✧ Classically cut garments rarely suit your unique sense of style. When classic proportions are fashionable, you will often search for clothing that is more distinctive.

✧ Most Aquarian women have a difficult time dressing in the style of the corporate world. Nothing bores you more than a traditional business suit.

✧ You can wear layered clothing but only when the layers are particularly light and airy. You shouldn't bulk up your silhouette with heavy fabrics. Avoid tweed altogether.

✧ Fabrics that drape well on your body appeal to you. When you wear a dress, you prefer it to be of a sheer fabric, like tulle, or of finely woven satin. Diaphanous fabrics have a special appeal to many Aquarius women.

✧ You should try to wear dresses more often. You have a highly social nature, and many of you enjoy going places where dressing up is appropriate. Always keep a party dress close at hand.

✧ High-tech materials suit you perfectly. You welcome revolutions in textile manufacturing, and you are often the first person to purchase something new. Many of you are especially fond of lightweight athletic fabrics.

✧ If you can't afford leather, try vinyl or PVC.

✧ You usually prefer to wear solid blocks of color rather than prints. You like the sharp contrast of bold color combinations, like a brightly colored top with a pair of black pants. However, glamorous prints appeal to you, too. Many Aquarius women profess a fondness for tropical prints.

✧ If your style is rather unorthodox, open your mind to the world around you and add some ethnic elements to your wardrobe.

✧ A bohemian look is simply a style that appears shocking or avant-garde to people who dress more conventionally. Play up the bohemian side of your nature by wearing what you like. Don't let anyone tell you how you should define your style.

✧ Because your zodiac sign rules over the cinema, old-style Hollywood glamour is especially attractive to your sense of style. People love to see what movie stars are wearing because their own lives are anything but glamorous. Therefore, glamour is essentially unconventional. Dressing in a glamorous style is one of the most eccentric ways to define your individuality.

✧ You can be inspired by science fiction. The costumes from *The Matrix* (1999) have a modern, high-tech look that may appeal to you.

✧ Your ruling planet can make you quite erratic. You may dress well on one day and not care what you wear on the next. Developing some consistency in the way you express yourself is important. Make a consistent effort to look your best.

✧ You probably don't spend a lot of money on designer labels, but you're not cheap, Aquarius. You just have different priorities than most people who buy designer clothing. With your extremely social nature, you would rather spend your money on cocktails and forget about the cocktail dress.

WHO TO WEAR

The Versace label suits unconventional Aquarius women ideally. Donatella Versace designs the most glamorous clothing in the world. Her sense of style is rooted deeply in the tradition of Hollywood glamour. She creates modern apparel that is tailor-made for television award shows and movie premieres. However, there is more to her designs than cinematic allure. She creates absolutely original clothes. Donatella Versace does her own thing. No other major designer acts so independently. When austere, minimal clothing is fashionable, she sends supermodels down the runway decked out like rock stars. When skirt lengths are hitting the floor, she's the only designer showing short dresses. She is a genuine eccentric, and most people only dream of being so outlandish. Electricity virtually crackles in the air at her shows, because the people who attend know they're in for a one-of-a-kind spectacle. You, Aquarius, are also one of a kind. Even if Versace doesn't appeal to you personally, you should be excited and inspired by the inventiveness of the world's most electrifying designer.

Another label you may find appealing is Betsey Johnson. She epitomizes the bohemian look, in both her signature designs and her own appearance. She creates youthful, eccentric clothing that appeals to a woman who wants to look different from everyone else. Like Donatella Versace, Betsey Johnson seems to do her own thing, unencumbered by the trends that constrain so many other designers. Another thing she has in common with Donatella Versace is that she makes very sexy clothes. But don't despair if you're not comfortable in sexy clothes, Aquarius. Take inspiration from these unique designers and find clothing that suits you. You are a unique woman, and no one knows what you should be wearing better than yourself.

WHAT TO AVOID

There are two basic types of badly dressed Aquarius women. The first type is the common Aquarius woman. She denies her unique nature by dressing in a style that can only be described as pedestrian. Her weak sun sign is to blame. The position of the sun in her chart thwarts her ability to express herself. She has a conservative bearing that defies her inherent eccentricity. Rather than allowing herself to celebrate her idiosyncrasies, she hides behind a mask of banality. Her incapacity for self-expression affects more than the way she dresses. She also leads a life that is far more ordinary than the life she dreams of. If you are one of these women, you must learn to express yourself. An Aquarian who refuses to recognize her individuality is like a ticking time bomb. It is not uncommon for her to blow up emotionally when the pressure of denial has become too much for her to bear. She can rebel against everything she has ever believed in, leaving others to wonder whether they really knew her at all. All of you Aquarians must learn to accept that self-expression is essential to your well-being. More is at stake than your looks.

The other type of badly dressed Aquarian is the trendy

Aquarius woman. She recognizes her sense of self-expression, but she ignores her originality. Instead of being the zodiac's most eccentric dresser, she is the zodiac's worst fashion victim. She dresses for shock value alone. She wears clothing that makes people grimace when they look her way. She believes that her own style is avant-garde. However, her so-called style comes in a shopping bag. If this scenario seems familiar to you, then you must learn to be original rather than derivative. If you have to buy a sense of style, you have no style. You're too smart to be a fashion victim, Aquarius. Put some thought into discovering what your style is; then you can set a few trends of your own.

HAIR AND MAKEUP

Your ruling planet likes change. Therefore, you should get in the habit of changing your look on a regular basis. Your hair is a great place to start. Many of you wear your hair short. As an air sign, you don't like to be weighed down with a heavy hairstyle. Even when you wear your hair long, you usually style it in a manner that is airy and voluminous. In fact, along with Leo women, Aquarians wear big hair better than anyone else. Regardless of the length of your hair, you must learn to style it creatively so that you can change it when you're in the mood. If you wear your hair long, try to avoid tying it back in a boring ponytail. Either style it or cut it off—it's as simple as that. Aquarians are always at their best when the styles are modern or futuristic. Any of you who were around in the early 1980s were likely delighted by the funky, futuristic hair that dominated the era. Get into the habit of coloring your hair, too. When you are required to conform to a standard of dress you dislike—in an office environment, for example—changing your hair color will allow you to express yourself. Wear any color that suits your complexion, and don't be afraid to try a daring color, like platinum blond.

You ought to have some daring colors in your makeup bag, too. Your natural eccentricity lets you get away with some rather unusual looks. Wear bright blues and greens. Try wearing corals and oranges, too. Cool colors generally suit Aquarian women better than warmer tones. But if your skin tone does not allow you to wear cool colors, you should choose shades that are colorful anyway. Avoid dull, earthy browns and fleshy pinks. Also, avoid wearing a lot of foundation. Because you are an air sign, you look your best with a light, fresh complexion. Try to avoid wearing glossy makeup and also avoid glossy, wet-looking hair products. However, if you aspire to be glamorous, you may need to go over the top with your makeup to create a visage that is both distinctive and dramatic. Put on some false eyelashes. Paint on a sexy beauty mark. Have some fun with your cosmetics, Aquarius, and never let anyone convince you that you don't look gorgeous.

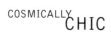
ACCESSORIES

Utilizing accessories to make your wardrobe more unique is an ideal way to cultivate some true Aquarian style. As mentioned before, Aquarius rules over the calves and ankles. Consequently, hosiery is an important part of the well-dressed Aquarius woman's wardrobe. It is likely that you own more hosiery than other women. Sheer panty hose looks especially attractive on you. Shimmery stockings suit you, too. If you are sensitive about the size or shape of your calves, remember that well-chosen hosiery can make almost anyone's legs look sexier. You probably own more socks than the average person, too. Many people don't even care if the socks they wear match, but Aquarians are rather picky about footwear. However, you may find that your eccentric nature is expressed most evidently in your eclectic shoe collection. You have quirky tastes, and you're just as likely to wear Ferragamos as Birkenstocks. But do yourself a favor, Aquarius. Choose the Ferragamos. Aquarius women also like boots. Boots are an important part of any well-dressed woman's wardrobe, but they should not replace the shoes in your closet entirely. Don't ever underestimate how great you can look in a pair of heels.

There are many other accessories that suit your sense of style. Jewelry made from semiprecious stones and rare minerals appeals to Aquarius women. Turquoise, coral, jade, and onyx all suit you well. Silver and platinum look better on you than gold. Diamonds look great on you, too, but you may choose to wear other precious stones simply because they are less commonly worn by other women. Sunglasses have a special appeal to the glamorous Aquarian woman. Women who walk around wearing sunglasses at night are commonly Aquarians. If you wear prescription glasses, you likely choose large, bold frames. You see no point in wearing eye makeup if you can't show off your artistry. You should try to carry handbags that are distinctive and unusual. You rarely spend an inordinate amount of money on designer purses. You prefer to have a dozen cheap purses rather than just one expensive bag with a label that means nothing to you. However, there is one accessory that Aquarians will spend a lot of money on. Many of you carry hand-held electronic organizers. But you don't carry them because they keep you organized, you carry them because you like gadgets. You can be a bit of a nerd, Aquarius. Don't try to fight it— just blame it on the stars!

SOME ADDITIONAL TIPS TO HELP YOU CREATE YOUR OWN COSMIC STYLE

- ✧ Most Aquarians love "Casual Friday." You despise business attire, and you welcome the chance to wear anything else.
- ✧ Aquarian women can be rather "indoorsy." Although you may practice good hygiene and possess exceptional

grooming skills, nothing will give your face a healthier glow than getting some fresh air.

✧ Very unnatural-looking nail color suits you well. Try blue, green, or silver. White nail polish looks especially attractive on you.

✧ A modern, sporty swimsuit will appeal to you.

✧ Your sleepwear and lingerie are often made from the latest and greatest new fabrics.

✧ Some astrologers claim that Aquarians normally marry later in life. It's not that you don't want to be married—you just don't want to put up with all the traditional fuss. Do yourself a favor and elope.

✧ A very modern wedding dress will suit you well. Avoid anything with ruffles or an inordinate amount of lace. Carry a few stems of bird-of-paradise flowers down the aisle.

✧ Light, airy fragrances suit you well. Try to shop around at more exclusive boutiques to find a perfume that is uncommon.

A FEW WOMEN WHO— FOR BETTER OR WORSE— EXEMPLIFY TRUE AQUARIUS STYLE

Chita Rivera: January 23

With her wiry body and electric stage presence, the actress Chita Rivera has an undeniably Aquarian air. Those qualities were never more evident than in *Sweet Charity* (1969). In false eyelashes and a big bouffant hairdo, Chita Rivera is the perfect example of 1960s Aquarius chic.

Oprah Winfrey: January 29

Oprah Winfrey looked gorgeous when she appeared on the cover of *Vogue* magazine. In a shot reminiscent of Hollywood studio photos of the 1940s, Oprah proved that no style enhances a well-dressed Aquarius woman more than over-the-top glamour.

Minnie Driver: January 31

Very few celebrities have made such a marvelous impression on the fashion press as Minnie Driver. She dresses exceptionally for every special event she attends. In typical Aquarius style, she has made herself look uncommon by being one of the few actresses in Hollywood who never looks bad.

Christina Ricci: February 12

Many women complain that only supermodels can wear designer clothing. But Christina Ricci looks as gorgeous as she wants to be in the glamorous designs of the Versace label. As an Aquarian she seems to delight in wearing clothing that other women would shy away from. Her friendship with Donatella Versace was written in the stars.

Dame Edna Everage: February 17

With her wisteria-colored hair and her one-of-kind couture gowns, Dame Edna Everage is the personification of Aquarian unconventional glamour. But despite her role as adviser to the British royal family, her attempts to get the Windsor women to dress in a more glamorous style have fallen upon deaf ears. Unfortunately, a gorgeous woman can give only so much caring and sharing.

PISCES
THE FISH

February 19–March 20

WHAT MAKES YOU
A PISCES

Poor Pisces! You're always last. Being the last sign of the zodiac shouldn't be a big deal, because the zodiac is a circle with no beginning and no end. Your sign is just placed last for the sake of convenience. However, some of you take offense at being put at the end, imagining there is some sort of conspiracy against you. You do have an overactive imagination, Pisces. You can be too sensitive, too. Sometimes when these factors combine, you can become completely irrational. You often allow your mind to wander into places you should never go. Left to your own devices, you can think way too deeply. In fact, you can become completely bewildered without ever leaving the familiar terrain of your own head. You may even prefer to live in your imagination instead of venturing into the real world. Doing this may put you in touch with your inner self, but it also puts you in touch with the darker side of your nature—and that scares you. You can thank your lucky stars that it doesn't scare everyone else away from you. Without your friends you could easily lose touch with the real world.

The reason you are somewhat unstable is your ruling planet, Neptune. Neptune was the Roman god of the deep, dark sea. He endows all Pisceans with depth. But he also endows you with a rather nebulous character. You have a difficult time putting your finger on what you really want from life. Many of you go with the flow, doing what other people tell you to do. You can find it difficult to define your own needs. Neptune also impairs your ability to make up your mind. However, his influence is not entirely negative. He also endows you with your best quality. The sea that Neptune rules over symbolizes creation, and Pisceans are remarkably creative. Your mind is like a bottomless ocean of ideas. You have the best imagination in the zodiac. Many of you are dreamers, and when your dreams are expressed through painting, writing, acting, singing, dancing, or any other creative endeavor, you can be wonderful artists. Although Neptune has bestowed on you an inability to define your own character, he has also given you the ability to express the undefinable.

In addition to being ruled by Neptune, Pisces is a mutable sign. The mutable quality makes you adaptable, but it also can make you incapable of forming an opinion. Pisces is also one of the water signs, along with Cancer and Scorpio. As a water sign, you can be terribly moody and far too introspective. When you're feeling blue, try to dress in a style that cheers you up. Or sit in front of the mirror and experiment with makeup in ridiculous ways until you make yourself laugh. Don't get stuck brooding over problems that exist only in your mind. Fashion can provide you an outlet that allows you to change your mood from bad to good. Like the old adage says, "Laughter is the best medicine."

It is the water element that gives you your extremely sensitive nature. In conjunction with Neptune, these factors blend to form typical Piscean characteristics. If you express these characteristics in a positive manner, you can be creative, imaginative, whimsical, sympathetic, and compassionate. If you express these characteristics negatively, you can be escapist, naive, vague, indecisive, and much too impressionable. Neptune can confuse you, Pisces. Therefore, you may not even recognize the difference between the positive and negative behavior you exhibit. But you must learn to show off the positive side of your character. In fact, you must learn to show off in general. You tend to live in your imagination, and many of you neglect to express yourselves externally. You may dream about being well-dressed, Pisces, but until you make an effort to look your best, your dreams will not come true.

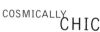
YOUR KEYWORD

Neptune impairs your ability to define your character. But rather than perceiving your indefinite nature as a fault, you should accept it as the one quality that makes you different from everyone else. *Indefinite* is your keyword, Pisces. Picture the water that represents your sign as clouds in the sky. As you stare into the sky, the clouds seem to constantly evolve into different shapes. Now imagine what those shapes could be. Almost everyone has played this game as a child, gazing up at the clouds with awe and wonder. You, Pisces, are like these clouds; you also can inspire awe and wonder with your presence. The well-dressed Pisces woman has an indefinite quality to her appearance that makes gazing at her enjoyable. She has a style that is whimsical, and she defies description because she seems to change before one's eyes. She is admired by everyone because she is a genuine free spirit. Like a cloud in the sky, she floats through life unconstrained, free from the boundaries that repress the rest of us.

YOUR THREE RULES TO DRESS BY

1: Imagine

The image of two fish swimming in different directions represents your sign. For this reason, Pisces is considered one of the dual signs of the zodiac. You ought to view this symbol as an accurate representation of your true nature. You are very whimsical, and you float through life unconstrained by conventionality. Because you are not grounded—many people have called you impractical—you can allow your boundless imagination to take you wherever you want to go. This imagination must be expressed in the way you dress. You don't fit into a specific mold, and dressing in a singular style defies your nature. Instead of trying to define yourself with a particular look, you need to imagine all the great looks you can be seen in. Don't adopt a definite style, Pisces. If you cultivate a boundless, imaginative style, there are no limits on how beautiful you can be.

2: Create

Your imagination is rooted in your innate creativity. Neptune endows you with an artistic, creative nature. However, many Pisces women live in a dreamworld. Rather than confront the realities of everyday life, you often retreat into the safe haven of your own mind. But sometimes this haven can seem more like an asylum because you can get swept away in your thoughts. For instance, it is well known that many Pisceans are hypochondriacs. They exhibit a single symptom of a harmless condition, but their overactive imaginations make them suspect the worst. All Pisces women must learn to use their imaginations in a more productive manner. A creative outlet is essential to your well-being. Fashion can be that outlet. By creating a new, exciting image for yourself every time you get dressed, you can burn off some of your more insidious mental energy rather than allowing it to get you into deep trouble. Creativity is therapeutic for you, Pisces.

3: Blur the Lines

Fashion has no definite rules for the well-dressed Pisces woman. There are no trends that she cannot transform to suit her own style, and there are no styles that she can't make trendy. There are no rules she cannot break, because her whimsical style can rewrite the rules of fashion. She is able to blur the lines between traditional and untraditional. She is able to erase the borders that define how gender is expressed through fashion. She can make good taste look like bad taste, and she can make bad taste become fashionable. The well-dressed Pisces woman has an indefinable quality to her sense of style. The conventions of fashion are inconsequential to her, yet she looks fabulous. She expresses herself with a deft attitude that makes her appear confident despite her rather insecure nature. She blurs the lines between perception and reality, making everyone believe that she's stylish. But only she knows the truth of the matter. She's not stylish—she's just good at clouding the issue.

SPECIFICS: WHAT TO WEAR

✧ It is likely that watery colors appeal to you. Colors that are indefinite also suit you well. When you see a color you can't accurately describe with a name, that is a Pisces color.

✧ Many introverted Pisces women wear dark colors regularly. Although black and navy blue may appeal to you, you should not get into the habit of wearing them exclusively. Dark colors can make you appear morose, and a lot more serious than you actually are.

✧ Odd mixes of color suit your sense of style. The last time there was a major Piscean influence upon fashion, wearing baby blue with chocolate brown became stylish. You can get away with any color combination. Wear what looks good on you.

✧ Odd mixes of fabrics suit you well. You should mix up styles, too. Wear leather pants with a sheer top. Put on a cowboy hat with a Hawaiian shirt. Or try wearing a tweed suit with pearls. You can create innovative outfits by mixing discordant elements from your closet. Fashion designers do this all the time to appear more innovative. You can do it because you're kind of crazy.

✧ Prints can play an important role in your wardrobe. Many people shy away from prints because trendy prints can date an outfit. But your sense of style has no time line, so don't worry about wearing something others consider dated. Just use your imagination, and wear what you own in a way that makes it appear new again.

✧ Certain fabrics will make you feel more comfortable than others. You prefer soft clothes to anything rigid. Knitwear appeals to you. Fluid fabrics suit you, too. You may wear heavier fabrics, but only when they are soft. Many Pisces women like to wear velvet.

✧ You should try to avoid wearing garments that need to be pressed. Pisces women don't like to iron. So instead of wearing wrinkly clothes, just wear clothes that don't get wrinkled.

✧ Many Pisces women have a dreamy, romantic nature. Consequently, many of you like wearing romantic-looking dresses.

✧ You likely express no preference between skirts and pants. However, as the zodiac's "gender bender," you wear pants well. You can look incredibly sexy in man-tailored garments.

✧ Many of you are fond of wearing men's jeans. You don't like the way women's jeans are cut.

✧ Wearing a very casual item with a rather spectacular garment will appeal to you. Put on a brocade smoking jacket over a pair of jeans. You'll get a thrill out of looking odd.

✧ Despite your propensity for gender bending, Pisces is widely recognized as the zodiac's most feminine sign. Girlish clothes suit you just as well as more masculine styles.

✧ You can get away with wearing things that other women would consider too feminine. Puffy sweaters, chiffon, feathers, fur, et cetera all suit you well. But try not to go overboard with a style that is obnoxiously cute. You'll appear much more attractive if you blur the lines between cute and sexy.

✧ Pisces rules over body art. Tattoos and piercings may appeal to you. Just remember that you have a whimsical nature, and a tattoo is a whim you'll have to live with.

✧ Your sign rules over illusion. Consequently, it also rules the profession of acting. Although you normally don't choose outfits for their dramatic appeal, costumelike clothing can suit you. When you have a special occasion to attend, don't be afraid to turn some heads in a gorgeous, cinematic costume.

✧ You spend money impulsively, so be careful you don't blow your rent money on a really great outfit.

WHO TO WEAR

Jean Paul Gaultier is the designer for you, Pisces. Gaultier has always astounded the fashion press with his remarkable imagination. But he also captured the attention of the world when he designed the costumes for Madonna's Blonde Ambition tour. His "cone bra" may be the most memorable outfit Madonna has ever worn. However, his pin-striped business suit with cutouts that showed off glimpses of Madonna's sexy lingerie was Piscean style at its best. Gaultier is the master of the mix. He has sent the sexiest models in the world down the runway in outfits inspired by nuns. He has sent men down the catwalk dressed like women. He has made gorgeous couture gowns out of run-of-the-mill fabrics, like tweed. He is a mad genius. You, Pisces, are a little crazy yourself. That is why the look of Gaultier was made just for you.

The Italian designers Domenico Dolce and Stefano Gabbana also create clothing that suits you ideally. More than any other label, Dolce & Gabbana blurs the line between good taste and bad. Like Jean Paul Gaultier, the charm of Dolce & Gabanna is in the untraditional mix of elements. However, there is something terribly romantic about the label. It is very feminine, despite the hard-edged "rock and roll" appearance of many of the garments. It is also rather showy, and much of it would look foolish worn by a more traditional woman. But you are not a traditional woman, Pisces. Showing off is something you must learn to do for the sake of your mental health. Your contemplative nature can be your downfall, because it constrains the expression of your imagination. You should be showing off clothing that expresses your creativity. The designs of both Jean Paul Gaultier and Dolce & Gabbana will allow you to do that.

WHAT TO AVOID

The worst-dressed Pisces woman is the introspective Pisces woman. She has no sense of the world around her, and she lives within the refuge of her own mind. As a result, she has no sense of self-expression. Fashion is fundamentally concerned with self-expression. It is an ideal outlet for an individual to manifest the most essential aspects of her character to the outer world. But the poorly dressed Pisces woman has her imagination and creativity stifled by her inability to express herself. If you are one of these introspective Pisces women, you must learn to live in the real world. Find yourself some friends who will help ground you. Force yourself to express your creativity through an art form. Learn to externalize your emotions. You have an impressionable personality, and you can easily be convinced to get out and enjoy life. So do it, Pisces. Put on something crazy and have some fun with your friends, before you get mired in the murky depths of your own mind.

Another type of badly dressed Pisces woman is the shapeless Pisces woman. Neptune bestows on you your indefinite nature. But an indefinite nature does not mean you should have no shape. When you are unhappy with the shape of your body, you may try to hide it under shapeless, baggy clothing because you are extremely sensitive. This also is a mistake. Baggy clothing can make you look worse by adding volume to your silhouette. There are many other ways to conceal your figure flaws. For instance, try emphasizing the aspects of your body you are pleased with. Wear garments that draw attention to all your best features. Most important, do something to achieve the body shape that would make you happy. Get to the gym, Pisces, and sweat out some of that anxiety before it consumes you entirely.

HAIR AND MAKEUP

You can have a lot of fun with makeup. Your imaginative, artistic nature makes you a great "painter." You should own a lot of makeup, and when you're bored or down in the dumps, you should play with your makeup just to see what you can accomplish. As mentioned before, you are essentially shapeless: You have an indefinite appearance that defies description. But you can use makeup to define yourself. Like an actress who never looks the same from one film to the next, you can be whoever you want to be. Just take the time to learn the necessary techniques. Makeup application is an art form, and it takes a great deal of practice. Find a friend who enjoys playing with cosmetics as much as you do. Together you can master the art of makeup. Glossy makeup suits you more than matte finishes. You may also be fond of products that add a sheen to your hair. Wet looks are a classic Pisces style. In addition, don't be restrained in your use of color, and don't be too timid to try new products. Furthermore, don't be afraid to leave your house with all that makeup on your face. People expect you to be a little foolish. After all, you are a Pisces.

Your hairstyle should be as versatile as your makeup palette. As a mutable sign, you keep up well with the trends. You can wear your hair fashionably long or stylishly short, but many of you like to wear it longer because long hair affords you even more styling versatility—at least that's what you tell yourself. Many of you, however, have long hair that hangs lifelessly from your head, because you just don't bother to style it. If this is the case, then cut it shorter. You'll look much better. In addition, get your hair cut often to keep it from looking shapeless and boring. Color changes also will help you keep your hair from looking boring. In fact, you should change your hair color frequently. Don't be constrained by the dictates of fashion, either. Dye your hair any color. Black, brown, blond, red, blue—it doesn't matter. Just express yourself in a manner that makes you feel happy about the way that you look.

ACCESSORIES

The well-dressed Pisces woman does not allow the conventions of fashion to inhibit her sense of style. She could wear an Hermès scarf one day and on the next pick a daisy from the roadside to put in her hair. She may carry her belongings around in an old lunch box or in a luxuriously beaded handbag. She could wear brightly colored Pucci leggings, or she could simply go bare-legged. No boundaries define her personal style. The one factor that characterizes her approach to wearing accessories is this: She owns a lot of accessories. She keeps her options open by keeping an entire wardrobe of accessories close at hand. It is never too late to start amassing a collection.

Shop at flea markets or rummage sales. Go to auctions and estate sales. Recognize that it takes more than a closet full of clothes to make a wardrobe.

Each zodiac sign rules over a certain region of the body. For you that area is the feet. Consequently, many Pisces women like shoes. However, Pisces also rules over addictions, and for that reason many Pisces women are shoe addicts. Some of you can't even walk past a shoe store without feeling the compulsion to go inside. You buy shoes religiously. You worship nice shoes, and you have a special place for them in your closet. You don't discriminate against any shoe styles. Pumps, sling-backs, mules, wing tips, sneakers, sandals—it doesn't matter what kinds of shoes they are, because you love them all. Although addictions are generally considered unhealthy, your obsession with shoes can be beneficial. As mentioned before, you can disregard your sense of self-expression entirely. But if you buy shoes obsessively, at least you do something to express yourself. It's better than doing nothing at all, Pisces.

SOME ADDITIONAL TIPS TO HELP YOU CREATE YOUR OWN COSMIC STYLE

✧ Don't wear a traditional gown to your wedding. Try something short, or—just for kicks—wear pants. Carry a bouquet of rare orchids down the aisle.

✧ Paint your nails in every color of the rainbow. Don't forget about your toenails, either.

✧ Because your sign rules over the feet, you should put extra effort into caring for your feet. Start by purchasing a pumice stone to scrape down your heels.

✧ Fruity fragrances suit you well. A hint of orange blossom in your perfume may appeal to you.

✧ Remember that "Casual Friday" does not mean "No Makeup Friday." Never make that mistake, Pisces.

✧ Slippery satin sleepwear appeals to you. Man-tailored pajamas in a typically feminine fabric suit your gender-bending style. Or try a baby-doll nightgown, since you can get away with cute clothes.

✧ Lingerie worn as outerwear can be an exciting addition to your wardrobe. The girdlelike bodysuit that Liza Minnelli wore in *Cabaret* (1972) looked terrific, especially with her high boots and bowler hat.

✧ Many of you love the beach, but more of you love the water. Be sure to chose swimwear that allows you to swim.

✧ Avoid excessive exposure to the sun. You're a worrier by nature, and the sun can quickly deepen those worry lines.

✧ Some Pisces women are exceptionally body-conscious. They worry about their shapeless form too much. They may even lose sleep simply deciding what to wear to the gym. The solution to this dilemma is to stop worrying and just get to the gym.

✧ Members of your sign are prone to depression. This is why you are obsessed with footwear—you hang your head too much. Get out of the habit of looking at your feet, Pisces. Walk proudly with your head up, and see all that the world has to offer you.

A FEW WOMEN WHO— FOR BETTER OR WORSE— EXEMPLIFY TRUE PISCES STYLE

Drew Barrymore: February 22

The actress Drew Barrymore has a whimsical style that suits her ideally. In typical Pisces fashion, she seems to delight in wearing anything and everything, unconstrained by the rules other women dress by. She is the epitome of Pisces style.

Elizabeth Taylor: February 27

Elizabeth Taylor shocked everyone when she emerged from a hospital stay with short, blond hair. The paparazzi swarmed around her during her first public appearance, seeming more interested in her new hairdo than in her clean bill of health. But she did look lovely. As a gorgeous Pisces woman, she can pull off any look.

Cyd Charisse: March 8

The classic Hollywood musical star Cyd Charisse never received the acclaim she deserved. In an era when women were soft and curvy, she had a gorgeous athletic body and legs that rippled with muscles. Her talent as a dancer was indisputable, but fifty years ago America wasn't ready for her gender-bending Pisces style.

Sharon Stone: March 10

Sharon Stone created a controversy when she appeared at an awards show dressed in a beautiful designer outfit over a T-shirt from the Gap. Of course she looked wonderful—she always does—but like any other well-dressed Pisces woman she proved that the secret to her sign's style is in the mix.

Glenn Close: March 19

The actress Glenn Close has a personal style that just blends into the background. She doesn't dress badly, but she wears boring, unimaginative outfits that don't do justice to her creative Pisces nature. She appeared to be having much more fun dressed as Cruella De Vil in *101 Dalmatians* (1996).